# Cardiology
## for the
## House Officer

**Second Edition**

# BOOKS IN THE HOUSE OFFICER SERIES

Burn Care for the House Officer

Cardiology for the House Officer, Second Edition

Clinical Pathology for the House Officer

Critical Care Medicine for the House Officer

Dermatology for the House Officer, Second Edition

Diabetes Mellitus for the House Officer

Diagnostic Radiology for the House Officer

Emergency Medicine for the House Officer

Emergency Psychiatry for the House Officer

Endocrinology for the House Officer

Hematology for the House Officer, Second Edition

Infectious Disease for the House Officer

Neurology for the House Officer, Third Edition

Neurosurgical Management for the House Officer

Obstetrics for the House Officer

Pediatric Cardiology for the House Officer

Pediatric Neurology for the House Officer, Second Edition

Psychiatry for the House Officer, Second Edition

Respiratory Medicine for the House Officer, Second Edition

Therapeutic Radiology for the House Officer

Vascular Surgery for the House Officer

# BOOKS IN THE CASE STUDIES FOR THE HOUSE OFFICER SERIES

Case Studies in Cardiology for the House Officer

Case Studies in Endocrinology for the House Officer

Case Studies in Neurology for the House Officer

Case Studies in Neurosurgery for the House Officer

Case Studies in Psychiatry for the House Officer

# Cardiology
# for the
# House Officer

## Second Edition

### Joel W. Heger, M. D.

*Getzen, Heger & Conrad Cardiology Group*
*Pasadena, California*

### James T. Niemann, M.D.

### J. Michael Criley, M. D.

*Harbor-UCLA Medical Center*
*UCLA School of Medicine, Department of Medicine*
*Division of Cardiology*
*Torrance, California*

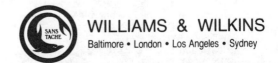

WILLIAMS & WILKINS
Baltimore • London • Los Angeles • Sydney

*Editor:* Nancy Collins
*Associate Editor:* Carol Eckhart
*Copy Editor:* Lindsay Edmunds
Design: JoAnne Janowiak
*Illustration Planning:* Wayne Hubbel
*Production:* Raymond E. Reter


Copyright © 1987
Williams & Wilkins
428 East Preston Street
Baltimore, MD 21202, U.S.A.

Accurate indications, adverse reactions, and dosage schedules for drugs are provided in this book, but it is possible that they may change. The reader is urged to review the package information data of the manufacturers of the medications mentioned.

*Printed in the United States of America*

First Edition, 1982

**Library of Congress Cataloging-in-Publication Data**

Cardiology for the house officer.
   Includes bibliographies and index.
   1. Heart—Diseases. 2. Cardiology. I. Heger, Joel W. [DNLM: 1. Cardiology—handbooks. WG 39 C267]
RC681.C178 1987      616.1′2      86-26781
ISBN 0-683-03947-4

88  89  90  91      10  9  8  7  6  5  4

# *Preface*

The first edition of **CARDIOLOGY FOR THE HOUSE OFFICER** was based on a loose-leaf syllabus originally developed for the housestaff and students on the Cardiology rotation at Harbor-UCLA Medical Center. The syllabus was frequently revised and updated in response to suggestions and criticisms from its readers.

The book was similarly field tested, but by a wider international audience, and this second edition incorporates suggestions made by its larger readership. In addition, there have been some remarkable changes in the practice of Cardiology in the past 5 years which necessitated extensive revisions. New diagnostic and therapeutic modalities have either been developed or have evolved from the experimental stage to everyday practice. Many chapters in this second edition bear little resemblance to their predecessors, with major changes in format, content, illustrations, and references.

The completion of this second edition could not have been accomplished in a timely manner without the selfless dedication of a number of individuals who gave many hours of their time to the task of updating and improving every aspect of the book. The editors would especially like to acknowledge the major contribution of Dr. Richard Haskell who is the author of the chapter on Pacemakers and who made a major contribution to the chapter on Echocardiography. In addition we are grateful to Dr. Milton P. Smith, Dr. Kenneth A. Narahara and Mr. Timothy Thigpen for their share of the scientific content, and Mrs. Ann Frick for the editorial aspects of this edition.

# Contents

# Chapter 1

# Basic Electrocardiography

The following chapter reviews common causes of abnormalities of atrial and ventricular depolarization and repolarization which may be recognized on the electrocardiogram (ECG). Arrhythmias may also produce changes in the morphology and/or duration of the ECG deflections and will be discussed in a separate chapter (Chapter 2).

It is beyond the scope of this text to provide a comprehensive presentation of basic electrocardiography and vectorcardiography. Discussion of electrophysiologic mechanisms underlying changes in the surface ECG are minimized in the following discussion and it is assumed that the house officer has a basic understanding of ECG vector analysis (calculating mean axes). Emphasis has been placed upon the differential diagnosis of QRS, ST, and T wave changes and providing the house officer with readily available ECG criteria for the diagnosis of commonly encountered ECG abnormalities. Comprehensive discussions of basic electrocardiography may be found in a number of texts(1-3).

## THE NORMAL ECG—WAVES, INTERVALS, AND SEGMENTS

The ECG is the surface representation of cardiac electrical activity. During myocardial depolarization and repolarization, deflections or waves are inscribed on the ECG. By convention, positive forces (electrical forces directed toward an ECG lead) produce upright deflections and negative forces (forces directed away from an ECG lead) are represented by downward deflections. The distances between deflections and waves are called segments and intervals, respectively.

## THE P WAVE

- Represents atrial depolarization.
- P wave duration (width) is a measure of the time required for depolarization to spread through the atria to the atrioventricular (AV) node. In the normal adult, maximum P wave duration is 0.10 sec.

- Mean frontal plane P wave axis (vector) is normally directed inferiorly and leftward (15-75°) and an upright deflection should be recorded in ECG leads I, II, and aVF.  A negative deflection is seen in aVR.  The P wave may be upright, isoelectric (flat), or inverted in III and aVL.
- Normal P wave amplitude is 0.5-2.5 mm (0.05-0.25 mV).

## THE PR INTERVAL

- Represents the time required for a supraventricular impulse to depolarize the atria, traverse the AV node, and enter the ventricular conduction system.
- Measured from the beginning of the P wave to the initial deflection of the QRS complex (Q or R wave) in the frontal plane lead with the longest PR interval.
- Normal PR interval is 0.12-0.20 sec in adults in sinus rhythm.  The PR interval normally shortens as heart rate increases and lengthens at slower heart rates.  First degree AV block is said to be present if the PR interval is >0.20 sec.  A PR interval of <0.12 sec may be seen as a normal variant, in hypocalcemia, with ventricular pre-excitation, and in ectopic junctional or low atrial rhythms.

## THE QRS COMPLEX

- Represents ventricular depolarization.
- Q wave--the first downward or negative deflection after the P wave and/or preceding the first upright deflection.
- R wave--the first positive deflection after a P wave.
- S wave--a negative deflection following an R wave.
- QS wave--a single downward deflection not preceded or followed by an upright deflection.
- R' wave--a second positive deflection after the R wave.
- Upper and lower case letters are frequently used to signify approximate voltages or amplitudes of R waves.
- QRS interval (duration)--an indication of intraventricular conduction time.  This measurement should be made in the frontal plane lead in which it is widest.  The normal valve in the adult is ≤0.10 sec.
- The mean frontal plane QRS vector in the normal adult is -30 to +110°.

## THE ST SEGMENT

- An isoelectric segment following ventricular depolarization and preceding ventricular repolarization.
- Measured from the end of the QRS complex to the beginning of the T wave.

- In contrast to the PR and QRS intervals, changes in the length of the ST segment are not as important as its deviation from baseline or the isoelectric point. The interval from the end of the T wave to the beginning of the P wave (TP interval) is usually taken as the isoelectric reference point. Elevation or depression of the ST segment by ±1 mm (0.1 mV) from the isoelectric baseline is considered "abnormal."

## THE T WAVE

- ECG representation of ventricular repolarization.
- T wave vector normally directed inferiorly and leftward.
- The T wave vector normally "tracks" with the QRS vector. If the QRS is predominantly negative in a frontal plane lead, an inverted T wave is usually seen and is not necessarily abnormal.
- An inverted (negative) T wave in V1 is considered normal. Inverted T waves in V2 and V3 may be normal in patients <30 years of age and in patients with "funnel chest" or "straight back" body habitus.

## THE QT INTERVAL

- Measured from the beginning of the QRS complex to the end of the T wave and represents duration of electrical systole. Mechanical systole usually begins during inscription of the QRS complex.
- This interval varies with heart rate. The normal QT interval, corrected for heart rate, is usually <.425 sec and is calculated by dividing the measured QT interval (in sec) by the square root of the R-R interval (in sec). The QT interval should be measured in the lead with the most clearly defined T wave.

## THE U WAVE

- A deflection following the T wave; electrophysiologic origin uncertain.
- U wave vector tracks with the T wave vector, i.e., polarity or direction similar.
- Amplitude greatest in precordial leads V2-V4.

### COMMONLY ENCOUNTERED ECG ABNORMALITIES

#### MISPLACED ECG LEADS

Figure 1.1 is an ECG tracing obtained from the same patient as in Figure 1.2. Note the difference in the axes of the P wave, QRS complex, and T wave recorded in the standard limb leads. This is a common technician error caused by reversing the right and left arm ECG leads (Figure 1.1). In switching the right and left arm leads, the frontal plane P, QRS, and T wave axes have been shifted rightward. Such frontal plane vector changes may also be seen in dextrocardia. However, in this example, the presence of a normal precordial (V1-V6) ECG eliminates dextrocardia as a differential possibility. With dextrocardia, horizontal plane QRS forces should be directed anteriorly and to the right, with decreasing R wave amplitude over the left precordium.

**Figure 1.1   Reversed ECG Leads**

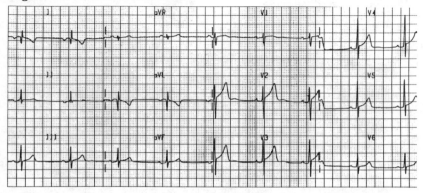

**Figure 1.2   Correct Lead Placement**

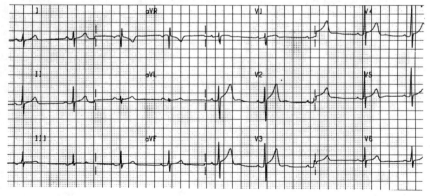

## EARLY REPOLARIZATION

Normal variant ST segment elevation may be noted in the precordial and limb leads. "Early repolarization" is the descriptive term applied to this ECG pattern. Whether accelerated subepicardial repolarization is actually responsible for the ECG variant is uncertain. ST segment elevation is most prominent in the lateral precordial leads (V4-V6). The T waves in these leads are characteristically broad-based, tall (usually >5 mm), and upright. The limb leads may also show some degree of ST elevation, but rarely greater than 2 mm. The early repolarization variant has been reported in all age groups, is more common in males, and is more prevalent in the black than the white population.

This variant may be confused with the ST segment changes noted during acute pericarditis. There are no universally accepted ECG criteria which accurately or absolutely distinguish between the two when a single ECG is examined(4,5). However, it has been suggested that the ratio of the ST segment amplitude to the T wave amplitude in lead V6 helps to distinguish the benign variant(6). In early repolarization, the ST/T ratio in V6 is generally less than 0.25. A ratio greater than 0.25 is usually seen in acute pericarditis. In the example (Figure 1.3) the ST/T ratio is 0.16.

## Figure 1.3  Early Repolarization

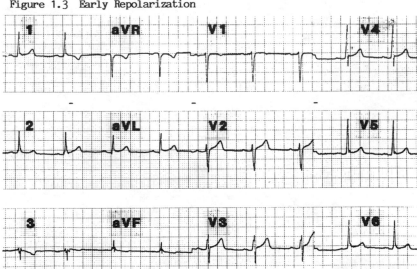

## PERICARDITIS

The ECG may be of considerable value in the diagnosis of pericarditis, especially if serial tracings are obtained(7). Evolutionary changes (stages) may be noted over several days.

Stage 1 (acute phase) (Figure 1.4)
- ST segment elevation in the precordial leads, especially V5 and V6, and in leads I and II.
- An isoelectric or depressed ST segment is commonly seen in V1.
- PR segment depression may be noted in leads II, aVF, and V4-V6.

Stage 2
- ST segment begins returning to baseline (isoelectric line).
- T wave amplitude decreases.

Stage 3
- ST segment isoelectric.
- T waves inverted in those leads previously showing ST segment elevation.

Stage 4
- Resolution of T wave changes.

Additional ECG abnormalities may be noted during pericarditis (see Chapter 14) and include arrhythmias, low-voltage QRS complexes (<5-mm R wave amplitude in limb leads), and electrical alternans.

## Figure 1.4  Pericarditis (acute phase)

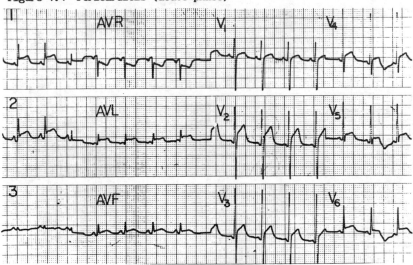

## THE ECG IN CHAMBER ENLARGEMENT

### ATRIAL ENLARGEMENT

Atrial enlargement may result from:
- Valvular heart disease (e.g., mitral stenosis).
- Pulmonary hypertension.
- Congenital heart disease (e.g., tricuspid atresia).
- Ventricular hypertrophy (e.g., systemic hypertension).

The initial portion of the P wave results from right atrial depolarization and the terminal portion from left atrial depolarization. The normal mean P vector is the sum of the vectors generated by both atria and is directed leftward and inferiorly. Atrial enlargement may alter the P wave magnitude, duration, or vector orientation.

An accurate ECG diagnosis of atrial enlargement is not always possible. There is considerable normal variation in P wave amplitude, duration, and morphology. Tachycardia alone may increase P wave amplitude. Although it is not always possible to diagnose left or right atrial enlargement electrocardiographically, the following criteria may be helpful:

### Right Atrial Enlargement (RAE)
- P wave amplitude of >2.5 mm in lead II.
- Frontal plane P wave vector shifted rightward (>+75°).
- Rarely noted as an isolated finding, i.e., most frequently associated with ECG criteria for right ventricular hypertrophy.

**Figure 1.5   RAE**

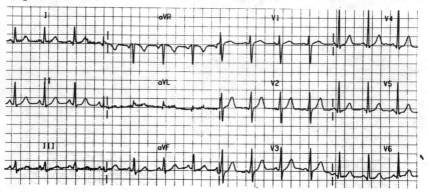

### Left Atrial Enlargement (LAE)
- P wave duration of ≥0.11 sec and P wave usually notched in lead II.
- Frontal plane P wave vector shifted leftward (0 to -30°)(terminal part of P wave may be negative in lead III and aVF).
- Biphasic P wave in lead V1 with wide, deep terminal component (≥ 0.04 sec in duration and 1 mm in depth).

## Figure 1.6  LAE

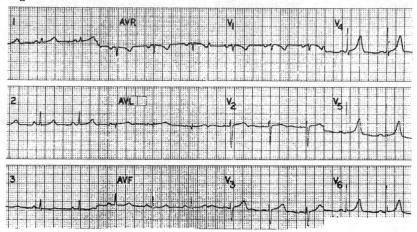

## LEFT VENTRICULAR HYPERTROPHY (LVH)

LVH manifests itself primarily as an increase in voltage (height of R wave) in those ECG leads which reflect left ventricular potentials.  The increase in voltage is due to an increase in muscle mass and surface area and/or the proximity of the dilated heart to the sensing ECG electrode (heart closer to chest wall).  The mean QRS vector tends to be rotated leftward and posteriorly.  LVH does not change the sequence of ventricular depolarization but may delay it (delayed onset of intrinsicoid deflection).  Repolarization may be altered--the left precordial leads may show depressed ST segments and inverted T waves--resulting in a left ventricular strain pattern.  The ECG diagnosis of LVH is based on voltage changes, ST-T wave alterations, axis deviations, and conduction delay (QRS duration of >0.08 sec but <0.12 sec).  A number of ECG criteria have been advanced, all of which have varying degrees of sensitivity and specificity.

### Common ECG Voltage Criteria for LVH in the Adult:

- Sum of S wave in V1 or V2 and R wave in V5 or V6 is >35 mm, **or**
- Sum of highest R and deepest S waves in precordial leads is >45 mm, **or**
- R wave in V6 of $\geq$18 mm, **or**
- R wave in a VL of $\geq$ 12 mm, **or**
- Sum of R wave in I and S wave in III is $\geq$ 16 mm, **or**
- R wave in I of $\geq$ 14 mm.

Limb lead criteria are less sensitive but highly specific.

## Point Score System for Diagnosis of LVH (Romhilt and Estes)(8)

Because LVH may affect the amplitude, axis, and duration of the QRS complex, as well as produce ST segment and T wave changes (down-sloping ST segment depression and asymmetric T wave inversion in V4-V6--strain pattern), a point score system was developed to improve diagnostic specificity. This commonly referenced point score system is less sensitive than QRS voltage criteria. With the current trend toward improved or high sensitivity to prompt the physician to seek more definitive or specific confirmation (echocardiography), the contemporary value of the noted criteria is questionable. The authors do not use this point system.

| Criteria | Points |
|---|---|
| 1. Amplitude of QRS | |
|     R in V5 or V6 $\geq$ 30 mm | |
|     S in V1 or V2 $\geq$ 30 mm | |
|     Largest R or S in limb leads $\geq$ 20 mm | |
|       If any one of the above present | 3 |
| 2. ST-T Strain Pattern | |
|     In the absence of digitalis RX | 3 |
|     Digitalis RX | 1 |
| 3. LAE Present | 3 |
| 4. Left Axis Deviation ($\leq$ -30$^\circ$) | 2 |
| 5. QRS Duration ($\geq$0.09 sec) | 1 |
| 6. Intrinsicoid QRS Deflection of $\geq$ 0.05 sec in V5 or V6 | 1 |

5 points or more - **definite LVH**

4 points or more - **probable LVH**

Figure 1.7   Left Ventricular Hypertrophy

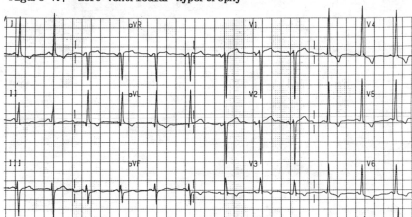

## RIGHT VENTRICULAR HYPERTROPHY (RVH)

The ECG diagnosis of RVH is less sensitive and less specific than that of left ventricular hypertrophy, and the ECG is frequently normal in the presence of RVH.  The following ECG abnormalities are suggestive of RVH:

- Right axis deviation (>+110° in an adult) in the absence of right bundle branch block (RBBB), left posterior inferior fascicular block, or anterolateral or inferior myocardial infarction.
- Dominant R wave ($\geq$7 mm) in lead V1 (may also be seen in right bundle branch block [RBBB], posterior myocardial infarction, Wolff-Parkinson-White [WPW] syndrome, and as a normal variant).
- R/S ratio in lead V1 of $\geq$1.0.
- R/S ratio in V5 or VG6 of $\leq$ 1.0.
- RSR pattern in lead V1 with a QRS duration of $\leq$.12.

The diagnosis of RVH is supported by the presence of RAE and/or right ventricular strain pattern (ST segment depression and T wave inversion in V1-V3).  The ECG diagnosis of RVH may be obscured if a RBBB is also present.

Figure 1.8   Right Ventricular Hypertrophy

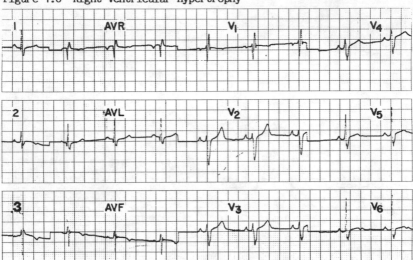

## COMBINED LVH AND RVH

The value of the ECG in the diagnosis of combined ventricular hypertrophy is limited. In many instances the ECG will demonstrate alterations suggesting hypertrophy of only one of the ventricles.

### ECG Criteria Suggestive of Combined Ventricular Hypertrophy:

- Voltage changes in the precordial leads "diagnostic" of both LVH and RVH.
- Voltage criteria for LVH plus:
  right axis deviation (>+110°), **or**
  R/S ratio in V1 of $\geq 1.0$, **or**
  $\geq 7$-mm R wave in V1, **or**
  deep S wave in V6, **or**
  right atrial enlargement and a vertical mean QRS axis.
- Voltage criteria for RVH plus:
  R/S ratio in V2-V4 and/or in two or more limb leads of nearly 1.0 (Katz-Wachtel sign), **or**
  large R waves in V5 or V6 with strain pattern and left atrial enlargement.

The ECG shown in Figure 1.9 demonstrates evidence of LVH (V6 R wave >18 mm and left atrial enlargement).   However, there is also right atrial enlargement and a right ventricular strain pattern is evident in the anterior precordial leads.   The frontal plane QRS axis is 90°--a more rightward axis would be expected with LVH alone.   The tracing is compatible with biatrial and biventricular hypertrophy.

**Figure 1.9   LVH and RVH (Precordial leads 1/2 standard)**

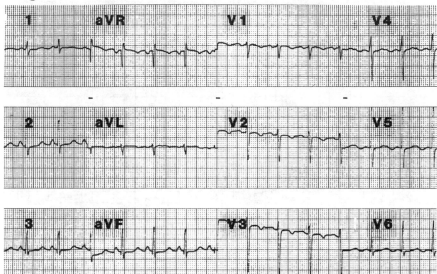

## THE ECG IN INTRAVENTRICULAR CONDUCTION DEFECTS

### RIGHT BUNDLE BRANCH BLOCK

Right bundle branch block is usually associated with organic heart disease (ischemic, rheumatic, congenital).   In RBBB, the sequence of ventricular activation is abnormal, resulting in a terminal QRS vector that is directed rightward and anteriorly (large R wave in V1, S wave in V6).   The cardiac vector is not significantly altered during the first 0.06 sec of ventricular depolarization.   The left ventricle is depolarized in a normal fashion, septal activation occurs from left to right, and the mean frontal plane QRS vector (axis) is usually normal. The site of block within the right bundle branch may be proximal or more peripheral.

## The ECG Criteria for the Diagnosis of RBBB Include:

- QRS duration of >0.12 sec in limb leads.
- Triphasic QRS complexes (RSR' pattern) in the anterior precordial leads (V1-V3).  The ST segment is often depressed and the T wave inverted in these leads.
- Wide S wave (0.25 sec in duration) in lateral precordial leads (V5, V6) and lead I.
- Normal time of onset of the intrinsicoid deflection in lead V6.

Associated RVH should be suspected if the secondary R wave in V1 is greater than 15 mm in amplitude or if there is right axis deviation of the mean frontal plane QRS vector.

**Figure 1.10   Right Bundle Branch Block**

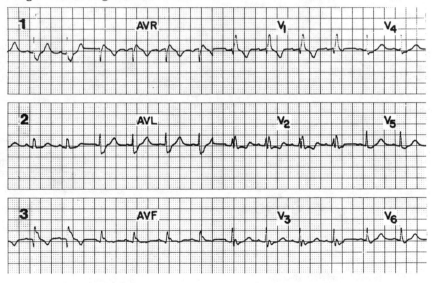

## LEFT BUNDLE BRANCH BLOCK

Left bundle branch block(LBBB) is almost always an indicator of organic heart disease.  In LBBB, the entire sequence of ventricular activation is abnormal, the primary abnormality being a change in the direction of the initial QRS vector.  Initial depolarization and the mean QRS vector are directed leftward and posteriorly.  Septal activation occurs from right to left.  There is also a change in the direction of repolarization--ST and T vectors rotate away from the mean QRS vector resulting in ST segment depression and T wave inversion in the lateral precordial leads, lead I and lead aVL.

The main left bundle branch divides into two major divisions (fascicles) soon after entering the interventricular septum--the left anterior superior fascicle and the left posterior inferior fascicle. Thus, LBBB may result from a lesion in the main left bundle, from simultaneous block in some portion of the anterior and posterior fascicles, or from peripheral block. The site(s) of block cannot be distinguished electrocardiographically.

## Electrocardiographic Criteria for the Diagnosis of LBBB Include:

- QRS duration of >0.12 sec.
- Large, broad, notched, or slurred R waves in the lateral precordial leads, lead I, and lead aVL. Q waves and S waves are characteristically absent, the ST segment depressed, and the T wave inverted in these leads.
- A small R wave precedes a deep S wave in leads II, III, and aVF.
- In most instances, left axis deviation (<-30°) is present. However, LBBB may be seen without left axis deviation.
- Initial R waves followed by deep S waves are present in the anterior precordial leads (V1-V3). The ST segment may be elevated in these leads.
- Onset of the intrinsicoid deflection is delayed in V6 but normal in V1.

From the description of the characteristic ECG findings, it should be apparent that a diagnosis of LVH or acute infarction is difficult in the presence of LBBB.

**Figure 1.11 Left Bundle Branch Block** (precordial leads 1/2 standard)

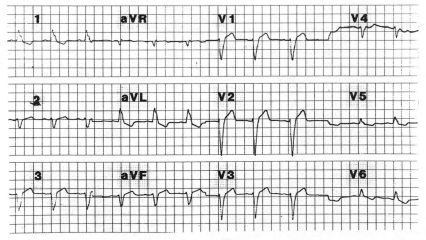

## THE FASCICULAR BLOCKS (HEMIBLOCKS)

The main left bundle can be considered to divide into two major divisions or fascicles soon after entering the interventricular septum-- the left anterior superior fascicle and the left posterior inferior fascicle.  Conduction delay in either fascicle (hemiblock) will alter the sequence of left ventricular depolarization and produce distinctive ECG changes.  Left anterior superior hemiblock, either alone or in association with AV nodal or right bundle branch conduction disturbance(s), is far more common than left posterior inferior hemiblock.  This disparity may be due to:  1) the greater length and smaller diameter of the anterior fascicle; 2) the location of the anterior superior fascicle within the turbulent outflow tract of the left ventricle; and/or 3) the single blood supply (left anterior descending coronary artery) of the anterior fascicle as compared to the dual blood supply of the posterior fascicle (LAD and right coronary artery).

### Left Anterior Superior Hemiblock (LASH)

If the anterior fascicle is blocked, the wave of depolarization will travel through the fibers of the posterior fascicle and then spread to the portions of the left ventricular myocardium normally activated by the anterior fascicle.  The sequence of left ventricular depolarization thus proceeds in an inferior to superior direction.  LASH may be caused by: coronary artery disease, valvular heart disease, congenital heart disease, cardiomyopathy, and myocarditis.

### ECG Criteria for the Diagnosis of LASH (Figure 1.12):

- Left axis deviation (mean frontal plane QRS axis of $\leq -45^{\circ}$).
- QRS duration usually $\leq 0.10$ sec.
- Small R waves in leads II, III, and aVF and small Q waves in leads I and aVF.
- Deep S waves in II, III, and aVF.
- Exclusion of other causes of left axis deviation:  body habitus, inferior myocardial infarction, hyperkalemia, ventricular pre-excitation, etc.

Figure 1.12  Left Anterior Superior Hemiblock (LASH)

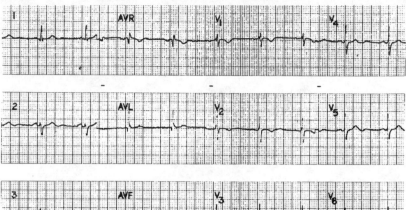

## Left Posterior Inferior Hemiblock (LPIH)

Ventricular activation proceeds in a superior to inferior direction. The mean frontal plane QRS axis will be directed inferiorly and rightward. LPIH is far less common than LASH, rarely occurs in the absence of associated AV nodal or right bundle branch conduction disturbances, and almost invariably indicates organic heart disease.

### ECG Criteria for the Diagnosis of LPIH:

- Right axis deviation (mean frontal plane QRS axis of >+110°).
- QRS duration of ≤0.10 sec.
- Small R waves in leads I and aVL and small Q waves in leads II, III, and aVF.
- Tall R waves in II, III, and aVF and deep S waves in I and aVL.
- Exclusion of other causes of right axis deviation: Chronic obstructive pulmonary disease (COPD), right ventricular enlargement, lateral myocardial infarction.

Figure 1.13  Left Posterior Inferior Hemiblock

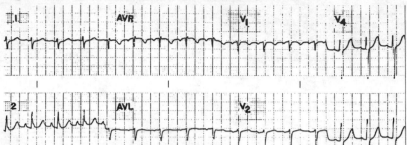

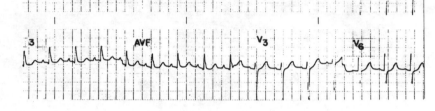

## BI- AND TRIFASCICULAR BLOCKS

Bifascicular block refers to the combination of RBBB with **either** left anterior superior **or** left posterior inferior fascicular block. Trifascicular block refers to the combination of RBBB with **either** left anterior **or** left posterior inferior fascicular block **and** incomplete AV block.  AV block may occur at the level of the AV node or more distally (bundle of His, main left bundle, or in the remaining fascicle).  The level of the AV block cannot be determined with the surface ECG--only a prolonged PR interval will be noted.  Figure 1.14 demonstrates RBBB, left anterior superior fascicular block, and first degree AV block.

Bi- and trifascicular block may be seen with:

- Coronary artery disease.
- Cardiomyopathy.
- Valvular heart disease, especially aortic.
- Lenegre's or Lev's disease--sclerodegenerative processes involving the cardiac conduction system.
- Cardiac surgery--repair of a ventricular septal defect or valve replacement.
- Myocarditis.

Although indicative of advanced conduction system disease, chronic bi- or trifascicular block alone is not an indication for permanent artificial cardiac pacing since long-term follow-up studies have not revealed a high incidence of complete heart block(9). Bi- or trifascicular block with clinical symptoms (syncope, dyspnea on exertion, etc.) due to documented bradyarrhythmias or complete heart block is an indication for artificial pacing.  Symptoms may be relieved, but the risk of sudden death will not be significantly affected.

**Figure 1.14   Trifascicular Block**

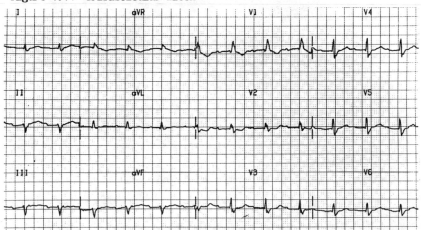

## THE ELECTROCARDIOGRAM IN ACUTE MYOCARDIAL INFARCTION

A single ECG is not the "gold standard" for the diagnosis of acute myocardial infarction (AMI).  The initial ECG may be nondiagnostic in 20 to 50% of cases of AMI(10).  The ECG diagnosis of AMI may be obscured or mimicked by a number of conditions(11).  The decision to admit a patient with chest pain to a coronary care unit should be based upon the patient's history and physical examination findings.

Serial ECGs during the acute phase of suspected AMI are of critical importance.  **Evolutionary ST segment and T wave changes during an acute transmural myocardial infarction** usually persist for only 1-2 days and are followed after a variable time period by T wave inversions in those ECG leads which showed ST elevation.  Persistent ST segment elevation beyond 2 weeks, especially in the anterior precordial leads, is a specific but insensitive index of a ventricular aneurysm, left ventricular dysfunction, and enhanced risk of sudden death(12). ST segment elevation persisting longer than 14 days after the acute event is usually permanent.

**ST segment elevation (especially in anterior precordial leads) is not diagnostic of transmural AMI as it may also be seen with:**

- LVH with strain.
- Left bundle branch block.
- Coronary artery spasm.
- Pericarditis.
- "Early repolarization."
- Hyperkalemia.
- Use of certain drugs (digoxin, tricyclic antidepressants).
- Cerebral vascular accident.
- Ventricular aneurysm.
- Hypothermia (Osborne waves).

**The ECG changes associated with nontransmural or subendocardial AMI are variable.** The ECG changes most commonly noted include:

- ST segment depression--down-sloping or "square wave" type of at least 1.0 mm.
- T wave inversion (Figure 1.13).
- ST segment depression **and** T wave inversion.

Characteristically, abnormal Q waves do not develop during the course of a nontransmural AMI. The ST-T wave changes may persist for a variable period of time but usually longer than 24 hours. The nonspecific character of these ECG changes often necessitates the use of ancillary studies (isoenzymes, radioisotopes) to confirm the diagnosis of myocardial necrosis. Patients suffering a subendocardial or nontransmural infarction may experience complications similar to those noted during transmural AMI and have a long-term prognosis not significantly different from patients with transmural necrosis(13).

**ST-T wave changes which simulate those of subendocardial infarction may also be noted in:**

- LVH with strain.
- The bundle branch blocks.
- Cardiomyopathies.
- WPW syndrome.
- Central nervous system disease.
- Late pericarditis.
- Electrolyte disturbances (especially hypokalemia).
- Association with the use of certain drugs.

The ECG is able to localize the site of infarction/injury with considerable accuracy based on which leads abnormal Q waves ($\geq$0.03 sec) or ST-T wave changes are noted.

Abnormal Q waves or ST-T wave changes in:

- II, III, aVF:  inferior wall infarction (Figure 1.16).
- V1-V3:  anteroseptal infarction (Figure 1.17).
- I, aVL, V4-V6:  lateral wall infarction (Figure 1.18).
- V1 or V2 to V6:  anterolateral infarction.

A large R wave and ST segment depression in leads V1 and V2 are indicative of infarction of the true posterior wall of the left ventricle. The large R wave and ST segment depressions noted in the anterior precordial leads are the surface ECG manifestations of posterior infarction/injury and may be viewed as "reciprocal" changes--if ECG leads were placed dorsally, characteristic Q waves and ST segment elevation would be noted. **Isolated posterior wall infarction is infrequent. This infarction pattern is most commonly seen in association with inferior wall infarction,** as these portions of myocardium share a common blood supply (right coronary artery in 90% of individuals).  Infarction of the inferior and/or posterior wall of the left ventricle is often complicated by infarction of the right ventricle.

**Figure 1.15  Subendocardial Infarction**

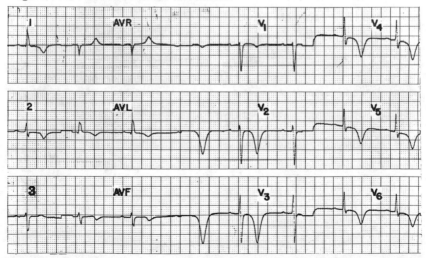

Figure 1.16   Inferior AMI

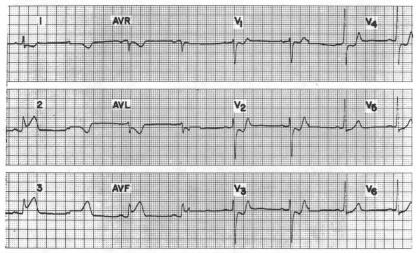

Figure 1.17   Anteroseptal AMI

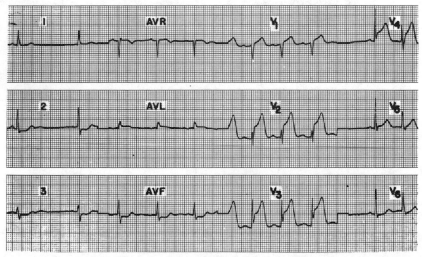

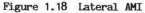

Figure 1.18  Lateral AMI

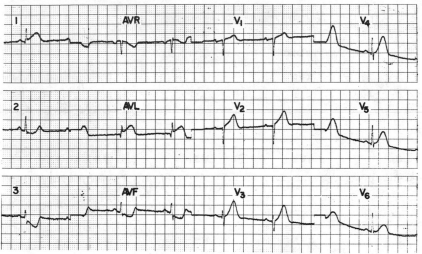

## ELECTROLYTES AND THE ELECTROCARDIOGRAM

Cardiac electrical activity results from the movement of various ions across the sarcolemma membrane. Changes in electrolyte concentrations may, therefore, alter depolarization and/or repolarization and produce ECG abnormalities(14).

### HYPERKALEMIA

1.  Serum potassium, 5.5–6.6 mEq/L.
    - Tall, peaked, narrow T waves in precordial leads.
    - Deep S wave in leads I and V6.
    - QRS complex usually normal.

2.  Serum potassium, 7.0–8.0 mEq/L (Figure 1.19).
    - QRS widening.
    - Slurring of both initial and terminal portions of the QRS.
    - ST segment elevation.
    - Low, wide P waves.
    - 1st and 2nd degree atrioventricular block.
    - Atrial arrest.
    - Bradycardia.

3. Serum potassium, >8.0 mEq/L.
   - Marked widening of QRS complex.
   - Distinct ST-T wave may not be noted.
   - High risk of ventricular fibrillation or asystole.

**Figure 1.19 Hyperkalemia**

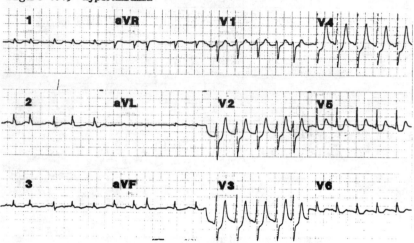

## HYPOKALEMIA

1. Serum potassium, 3.0-3.5 mEq/L.
   - ECG may be normal.
   - If ECG changes are present, they are most prominent in the anterior precordial leads V2 and V3 and consist of T wave flattening and the appearance of U waves.
   - QT interval and QRS duration normal.

2. Serum potassium, 2.7-3.0 mEq/L (Figure 1.20).
   - U waves become taller and T waves become smaller but do not invert.
   - The ratio of the amplitude of the U wave to the amplitude of T wave frequently exceeds 1.0 in V2 or V3.

3. Serum potassium, <2.6 mEq/L.
   - Almost always accompanied by ECG changes.
   - ST segment depression associated with tall U waves and low-amplitude T waves.

- QT interval normal, but accurate measurement may be difficult due to the close proximity of the U wave. The U wave is usually smallest in lead aVL and this lead should be used to determine the QT interval.
- QRS duration rarely affected in adults.

**Figure 1.20 Hypokalemia**

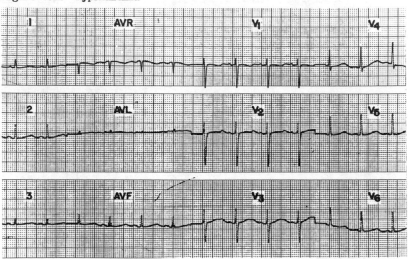

## HYPERCALCEMIA

- Slight increase in QRS duration.
- ST segment short or absent.
- Corrected QT interval shortened.
- PR interval may be prolonged.
- T wave amplitude and duration usually normal.
- U wave amplitude may be normal or slightly increased.

## HYPOCALCEMIA (Figure 1.21)

- Slight decrease in QRS duration.
- ST segment lengthened and corrected QT interval prolonged.
- PR interval may be shortened.
- T waves may become flat or inverted in severe hypocalcemia.

Figure 1.21   Hypocalcemia

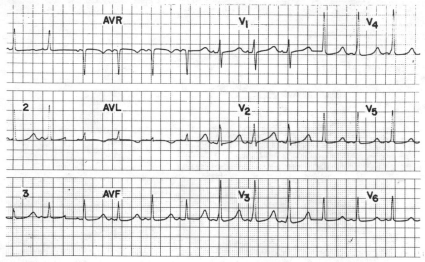

## HYPO- or HYPERNATREMIA

- Effects of changes in serum sodium cannot be detected electrocardiographically.

## HYPO- or HYPERMAGNESIUM

- Marked magnesium deficiency is usually associated with potassium depletion and the ECG demonstrates the characteristic changes of hypokalemia. Ventricular arrhythmias may be present.
- Hypermagnesium is uncommon clinically and is usually encountered in patients with uremia who often have other electrolyte disturbances (hypocalcemia, hyperkalemia) which produce ECG changes.
- It is uncertain if changes in body magnesium alone affect the surface ECG.

### NONCARDIAC DRUGS AND THE ECG

Commonly used inotropic (digoxin) and antiarrhythmic (quinidine, procainamide) drugs produce well-defined repolarization changes which can be recognized on the surface ECG. Noncardiac drugs can also produce significant ECG changes which may be confused with organic cardiac disease(15). The phenothiazines and tricyclic antidepressants are frequently used in clinical practice and may produce a number of "benign" or significant ECG changes. These drugs share a number of electrophysiologic effects with the group I antiarrhythmic drugs (e.g., quinidine) and thus have a direct effect upon the cardiac action potential. These drugs also possess variable anticholinergic properties and can affect the heart indirectly.

## PHENOTHIAZINES

ECG abnormalities may be noted in 50% of patients receiving "therapeutic" doses of these agents and there is no definite relationship between dose, serum level, or duration of therapy and the incidence of ECG abnormalities. Thorazine and Mellaril have been most frequently reported to produce ECG changes. Life-threatening arrhythmias have been reported following toxic (suicidal) ingestions. Characteristic ECG changes include:

Therapeutic doses (mimics hypokalemia)
- Prominent U waves.
- Low-amplitude T waves or T wave inversion.
- ST segment depression.
- Prolonged QT interval.

Toxic doses
- Prolonged QT interval and QRS duration.
- AV and intraventricular conduction delay.
- Increased automaticity.
- Ventricular arrhythmias due to re-entry.

## TRICYCLIC ANTIDEPRESSANTS

Therapeutic doses usually do not produce ECG changes except sinus tachycardia during the early phase of therapy (parasympatholytic effect). In toxic doses, ECG changes similar to those noted with toxic doses of a phenothiazine are usually present and are due to a direct effect of these drugs on the myocardium. Additional characteristic findings include rightward deviation of terminal QRS forces and anterior rotation of the ST segment vector.

### THE ECG IN CENTRAL NERVOUS SYSTEM DISEASE

Central nervous system (CNS) lesions, particularly subarachnoid hemorrhage, intracerebral hemorrhage, and infarction (stroke), may produce striking ECG repolarization abnormalities(16). These alterations most commonly take the form of diffuse, deep, wide, blunted T wave inversions and QT prolongation; U waves may also be prominent. The exact incidence of ECG changes in CNS hemorrhage or infarction is undetermined but appears to be more common with frontal lobe lesions. These functional repolarization changes are felt to be due to heightened cerebrocardiac autonomic stimuli.

## ARTIFICIAL CARDIAC PACEMAKER

The tip of a transvenous ventricular pacing catheter should lie in the apex of the right ventricle. Electrocardiographically, the mean QRS vector of paced complexes will depend upon the point of electrical stimulation of the myocardium. If the catheter tip is properly positioned, the mean QRS vector of paced complexes should be directed superiorly and posteriorly, resulting in:

- large, wide QRS complexes with a dominant R wave in leads I, aVL, and commonly in V6.
- large, negative deflections (QS waves) in leads II, III, aVF, and V1-V3.

The ECG pattern thus mimics that of a left bundle branch block with left axis deviation.

In Figure 1.22, each QRS complex is preceded by a pacemaker stimulus artifact ("spike"), which is seen best in leads I and aVL and the precordial leads. AV dissociation is also present. Small pacemaker spikes, as in Figure 1.22, are typical of a bipolar pacemaker. Unipolar pacemakers characteristically produce larger ECG spikes because the electrodes are farther apart and the generated current is transmitted through a greater amount of body tissue.

**Figure 1.22 Paced Rhythm**

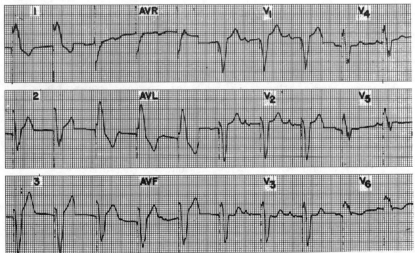

## WOLFF-PARKINSON-WHITE SYNDROME

Wolff-Parkinson-White (WPW) syndrome is a form of anomalous AV conduction or pre-excitation(17).  Ventricular **pre-excitation** is said to exist when conduction of a supraventricular impulse to the ventricular myocardium occurs via accessory pathways which bypass the AV node. Conduction via an accessory pathway in WPW permits premature activation of ventricular myocardium.  Pre-excitation can occur through a number of anatomic pathways.  In classic WPW syndrome, a sinus impulse is conducted through the **bundle of Kent**, which bypasses the AV node, and initiates activation of the ipsilateral ventricle.  A short PR interval and an initial slurring (**delta wave**) during the inscription of the QRS complex result.  The bypass tract is capable of bidirectional conduction, and re-entrant tachyarrhythmias (see Chapter 2) are a feature of this syndrome.

Recent electrophysiologic studies in humans, including epicardial ECG monitoring ("mapping") during open heart surgery, have yielded a great deal of information regarding sites of bypass tracts and their electrophysiologic behavior.  A new classification for the WPW syndrome has been proposed and is based on the anatomic site of the bypass tract: 1) right sided; 2) left sided; or 3) septal (within the membranous intraventricular septum).

### ECG Criteria for the Diagnosis of WPW Syndrome:

- Short PR interval (<0.12 sec).
- Normal P wave vector (to exclude junctional rhythm).
- Presence of a delta wave--slurring or notching of first portion of the QRS complex.
- QRS duration greater than 0.10 sec.

### Clinical Significance of the WPW Syndrome:

- High incidence of tachyarrhythmias (usually re-entrant mechanism--40-80% of patients).
- Frequently associated with organic heart disease (30-40% of cases). Disorders commonly associated with WPW syndrome include: atrial septal defect, mitral valve prolapse, hypertrophic cardiomyopathy, and Epstein's anomaly.
- ECG patterns may simulate other disease processes--myocardial infarction or ventricular hypertrophy.
- Antegrade conduction via the bypass tract and retrograde conduction through the AV node may produce regular tachyarrhythmias with wide QRS complexes mimicking ventricular tachycardia.

**Figure 1.23  Pre-excitation**

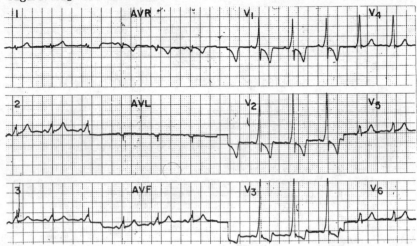

## REFERENCES

1.  Cooksey JD, Dunn M, Massie E:  Clinical Vectorcardiography and Electrocardiography, 2nd Edition, Chicago, Year Book Medical Publishers, Inc., 1977.

2.  Friedman HH:  Diagnostic electrocardiography and vectorcardiography, 2nd Edition, San Francisco, McGraw-Hill Book Co., 1977.

3.  Goldman MJ:  Principles of Clinical Electrocardiography, 8th Edition, Los Altos, Calif., Lange Medical Publications, 1973.

4.  Spodick DH:  Differential characteristics of the electrocardiogram in early polarization and acute pericarditis.  N Engl J Med 295:523, 1976.

5.  Wanner WR, Schaal SF, Bashore TM, et al.:  Repolarization variant vs acute pericarditis. A prospective electrocardiographic and echocardiographic evaluation.  Chest 83:180, 1983.

6.  Ginzton LE, Laks MM: The differential diagnosis of acute pericarditis from the normal variant:  New electrocardiographic criteria.  Circulation 65:1004, 1982.

7.  Spodick DH:  Electrocardiogram in acute pericarditis.  Distributions of morphologic and axial changes by stages.  Am J Cardiol 33:470, 1974.

8.  Romhilt DW, Estes EH:  Point score system for the ECG diagnosis of left ventricular hypertrophy.  Am Heart J 75:752, 1968.

9.  McAnulty JH, Rahimtoola SH:  Chronic bundle-branch block. Clinical significance and management.  JAMA 246:2202, 1981.

10.  McGuinnes JB, Begg TB, Semple T:  First electrocardiogram in recent myocardial infarction.  Br Med J 2:449, 1976.

11.  Goldberger AL:  ECG simulators of myocardial infarction. Pathophysiology and differential diagnosis of pseudo-infarct q wave patterns (Part I).  PACE 5:106, 1982.  Pathophysiology and differential diagnosis of pseudo-infarction ST-T patterns (Part II).  PACE 5:414, 1982.

12.  Arvan S, Varat MA:  Persistent ST-segment elevation and left ventricular wall abnormalities:  A 2-dimensional echocardiographic study.  Am J Cardiol 53:1542, 1984.

13.  Moreno P, Schocken DD:  Non-Q wave myocardial infarction. Pathophysiology and prognostic implications.  Chest 86:905, 1984.

14.  Surawicz B:  Electrolytes and the electrocardiogram.  Postgrad Med 55:123, 1974.

15.  Duke M:  The effects of drugs on the electrocardiogram—a reference chart.  Heart and Lung 10:698, 1981.

16.  Abildskov JA, Millar K, Burgess MJ, et al.:  The electrocardiogram and the central nervous system.  Prog Cardiovasc Dis 13:210, 1970.

17.  Mandel WJ, Yamaguchi I, Laks MM:  Syndromes of accelerated conduction.  Adv Cardiol 22:80, 1978.

# Chapter 2

# Arrhythmias:
# Recognition and Management

The following chapter reviews the basic rules and principles of arrhythmia interpretation. Examples and descriptions of common arrhythmias are provided and a basic approach to therapy is included for each arrhythmia.

## BASIC RULES FOR RHYTHM INTERPRETATION

1. Identify atrial activity--P waves

   - Is there evidence of atrial depolarization, i.e., are P waves present?

   - If so, do they represent normal P waves, ectopic P' waves, the F waves of atrial flutter, or the fibrillatory waves of atrial fibrillation?

   - Do the atria depolarize in an "anterograde" (upright P in lead II) in a "retrograde" (negative P in lead II) manner?

   - Are all P waves in a single lead of similar morphology, i.e., do all P waves look the same?

   - What is the atrial rate?  Is it regular or irregular?

2. Identify ventricular activity--QRS complexes

   - Does ventricular depolarization arise from a supraventricular focus; i.e., is the QRS of normal duration (<0.10 sec)?

   - If the QRS is broad, is it the result of aberrant ventricular conduction, or an ectopic ventricular focus?

   - What is the ventricular rate?  Is it regular or irregular?

3.   Evaluate atrioventricular (AV) conduction--analyze the relationship
     between the P wave and the QRS.

   - Is each P wave related to a QRS?   If the PR interval is <0.10 sec or
     >0.40 sec, the P wave is unlikely to have "produced" the ensuing QRS
     complex.

   - Is each P wave conducted to the ventricles (1:1 AV conduction)?

   - Is the speed of AV conduction (the PR interval) normal?

   - Is there any evidence of group beating (Wenckebach)?

## SUPRAVENTRICULAR ARRHYTHMIAS

### SINUS BRADYCARDIA

Description:

     Sinus bradycardia (Figure 2.1) is the result of a decrease in the
normal rate of discharge of the sinoatrial (SA) node.   The atrial rate (P
wave frequency) is less than 60/min, but atrial depolarization is normal
(i.e., the P wave vector is directed inferiorly and leftward and upright P
waves are seen in leads II, III, and aVF).   The P-to-P interval is regular
and each P wave is followed by a QRS complex of normal duration (1:1 AV
conduction).   The PR interval is fixed or constant.   In the setting of an
underlying interventricular conduction defect, QRS complexes may be of
prolonged duration (>0.10 sec).

Figure 2.1   Sinus Bradycardia

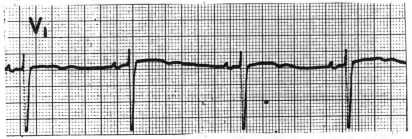

Causes:

- **Normal.**  Increased vagal tone in the conditioned athlete.

- **Pathologic.**
    Intrinsic sinus node disease--sick sinus syndrome.
    Increased vagal tone--inferior myocardial infarction, vasovagal
        response.
    Drug toxicity--beta-adrenergic blockade, calcium channel
        blockade, organophosphate poisoning.

**Therapy:**

Therapy is dictated by the clinical circumstances in which sinus bradycardia is noted.  Acute therapy is always indicated if hemodynamic compromise/hypoperfusion is present.  In the setting of acute inferior myocardial infarction, acute therapy is also indicated if ventricular arrhythmias (ventricular escape beats or rhythms or premature ventricular contractions) are present.

**Atropine Sulfate.**  Atropine is the drug of choice if sinus bradycardia is pathologic and associated with hypoperfusion.  It is most effective if symptomatic bradycardia is the result of acute inferior myocardial infarction, a vasovagal response, or cholinergic drug toxicity.  The drug should be administered intravenously, and 0.5-mg boluses administered at 5-min intervals (to a total dose of 2.0 mg) are recommended(1).  In the setting of acute inferior myocardial infarction, a total dose of about 1 mg is usually successful in increasing the sinus rate(2).  Atropine is of limited value in managing hemodynamically significant bradyarrhythmias associated with the sick sinus syndrome(3).  It is unlikely to increase heart rate in the setting of drug toxicity due to beta-adrenergic or calcium channel blockade.  Excessive use of atropine may result in sinus tachycardia and an increase in myocardial oxygen demand(2).  This complication is of particular concern in the patient with atherosclerotic coronary artery disease (CAD).

**Isoproterenol Hydrochloride.**  Isoproterenol (Isuprel) is a pure beta agonist.  It will produce a decrease in peripheral arterial tone and arterial pressure will fall if its use does not produce an increase in cardiac output (via beta-1-mediated increased heart rate or improved contractility).  Isoproterenol should be used with caution in the setting of acute infarction since it will increase myocardial oxygen demand that may not be met by an increase in myocardial oxygen supply(1).  In addition, it may be arrhythmogenic and is of limited value in the setting of beta-adrenergic blocker toxicity(4).  Isoproterenol is most commonly used to treat hemodynamically significant bradyarrhythmias unresponsive to atropine.  It should be administered as a continuous intravenous infusion at an infusion rate of 2-5 mu/min titrated to the hemodynamic response.

**- Artificial Cardiac Pacing.** If pharmacologic therapy is unsuccessful, temporary artificial cardiac pacing should be instituted as soon as possible.

**- Calcium Chloride.** May be of value in the setting of calcium channel blocker toxicity. An IV dose of 100-500 mg of a 10% calcium chloride solution may reverse peripheral dilation associated with calcium blocker toxicity, but may not increase heart rate(5).

**- Glucagon.** May be the drug of choice in the setting of beta blocker toxicity(4). An IV bolus dose of 2-4 mg is recommended. Vomiting may occur and the means to prevent aspiration should be available.

## SINUS TACHYCARDIA

### Description:

Sinus tachycardia (Figure 2.2) results from an increased rate of discharge of the sinus node and is usually a physiologic response to a demand for an increase in cardiac output.   The atrial rate is 100-160/min, and the P-to-P interval is regular.   P waves are upright in leads II, III, and aVF (normal atrial depolarization and P wave vector).   Each P wave is usually followed by a normal QRS complex (1:1 AV conduction).   However, second degree atrioventricular block may occur, and QRS duration may be prolonged in patients with an interventricular conduction defect (fixed bundle branch block, rate-related bundle branch block, aberrant ventricular conduction).   Carotid sinus massage or a properly performed Valsalva maneuver may transiently slow the SA node discharge rate and be of value in diagnosis in confusing cases (e.g., sinus discharge rate of 140-160/min with 1:1 AV conduction, which can be confused with atrial flutter with a 2:1 AV block or re-entrant or automatic atrial supraventricular tachyarrhythmias).   These maneuvers will not terminate this rhythm and may have no effect.

**Figure 2.2 Sinus Tachycardia**

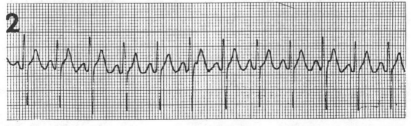

## Causes:

Causes include pain, anxiety, hypovolemia, left ventricular dysfunction, fever, pulmonary embolism, thyrotoxicosis, drug toxicity (e.g., cocaine, amphetamines, tricyclic antidepressants, anticholinergic drugs), drug withdrawal (e.g., narcotics, alcohol), and autonomic insufficiency.

## Therapy:

Sinus tachycardia is a physiologic response of the sympathetic nervous system to meet a demand for an increase in cardiac output. Therapy will be effective only if the physiologic stimulus for the cardiac response can be defined. Therapy should, therefore, be directed toward correction of the physiologic stimulus. A complete history and physical examination will yield the most valuable information and will most often define the cause.

If the history and physical examination fail to yield a physiologic stimulus for this rhythm disturbance, consider:

- **Pulmonary Embolism.** Sinus tachycardia is the most frequent cardiac response to this physiologic insult, and the clinical diagnosis of pulmonary embolism is imprecise.

- **Hyperthyroidism.** Sinus tachycardia is frequently associated with this endocrine abnormality, and most other physical findings are nonspecific.

- **Hypovolemia.** Postural vital signs should be obtained during careful monitoring.

## SINUS ARRHYTHMIA

## Description:

This irregular supraventricular arrhythmia (Figure 2.3) results from phasic alterations in vagal tone and is reflected by a gradual increase and decrease in the rate of sinus node discharge. The reflex arc is initiated by normal respiration. Inspiration decreases vagal tone and produces an increase in the rate of SA discharge. Expiration results in increased vagal tone and a decrease in the rate of SA discharge. This is a normal phenomenon, especially in children and young adults. It may be accentuated by drugs (digoxin) in the elderly. Atrial depolarization is normal (upright P waves in leads II, III, and aVF) but irregular; there is a gradual increase and decrease in the P-P interval. The minimum difference between the longest and shortest P-P interval is usually 0.16 sec. The PR interval remains constant, and each P wave is followed by a QRS complex. The resultant rhythm is irregularly irregular and must be differentiated from other causes of an irregularly irregular rhythm (see Atrial Fibrillation).

Figure 2.3 Sinus Arrhythmia

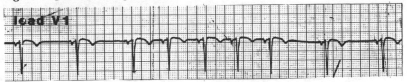

Causes:

Physiologic   drug-induced (e.g., digoxin); marked sinus arrhythmia; may be a manifestation of the sick sinus syndrome.

Therapy:

The arrhythmia is physiologic and requires no therapy.   Confusion may arise when it is mistaken for another rhythm disturbance.

## PREMATURE ATRIAL CONTRACTIONS (PACs)

Description:

A PAC is an electrical impulse which originates within the atrial myocardium but outside the SA node.   It is premature (i.e., occurring before the next expected sinus discharge) and produces atrial depolarization and a P' wave which differs in morphology from P waves of sinus node origin.   A PAC usually depolarizes the SA node because the SA node is not "electrically isolated."   The interval between the sinus P waves preceding and following a PAC is less than twice the normal P-P interval, resulting in a pause that is not fully compensatory.   PACs originating from the same focus (unifocal PACs) have morphologically similar P' waves and a fixed coupling interval (the P-P' interval).   When PACs are multifocal, P' waves differ in morphology and the coupling interval varies.

A PAC may be conducted normally through the AV node and ventricles. However, it may be conducted with partial AV block (PR interval greater than 0.20 sec) or be completely blocked (nonconducted PAC) at the level of the AV node if the coupling interval is short (P' wave occurs close to T wave).   Incomplete block and slow conduction at the bundle branch level may result in "aberrant" ventricular conduction (see Aberrant Ventricular Conduction).

Two PACs are demonstrated in Figure 2.4. The ectopic P' waves are marked with arrowheads. The P' waves occur earlier than the next expected sinus P wave. The P'R interval is longer than the PR interval of normal sinus beats (beats 1, 2, 4, 5, and 7), indicating conduction delay. The P' waves differ in morphology and the ectopic coupling interval also varies--this suggests that these PACs are of multifocal origin.

**Figure 2.4 Premature Atrial Contractions (PACs)**

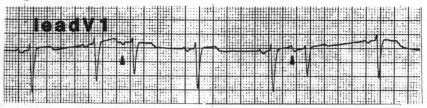

## Causes:

Causes include increased circulating catecholamines, drug toxicity (e.g., theophylline, sympathomimetics), and pericarditis (rarely).

## Therapy:

If frequent PACs are associated with symptomatic episodes of paroxysmal supraventricular tachyarrhythmias, quinidine, procainamide, or beta blockers can be used to decrease atrial automaticity.

## MULTIFOCAL ATRIAL TACHYCARDIA (MAT)

### Description:

MAT is an ectopic, repetitive atrial arrhythmia which results from enhanced atrial automaticity; it frequently precedes the onset of atrial fibrillation(6,7). Ectopic atrial electrical activity from three or more foci produces an irregular atrial rate as well as an irregular ventricular rate. The atrial rate is usually 100-180/min with a varying P-P interval. The PR interval usually varies from beat to beat. The ventricular rate is also irregular (varying R-R interval). Ectopic P' waves (best seen in leads II, III, and aVF) vary in morphology. MAT can be confidently diagnosed if three consecutive P waves of different morphology at a rate >100/min are identified in a single lead(8).

An episode of MAT is shown in Figure 2.5. Three consecutive ectopic P' waves are indicated by arrows. The P-P, PR, and R-R intervals vary in an irregularly irregular fashion.

## Figure 2.5 Multifocal Atrial Tachycardia

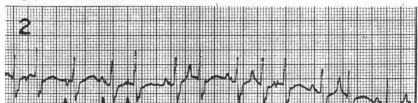

### Causes:

MAT is most commonly encountered in patients with chronic obstructive lung disease and acute respiratory failure or patients with severe left ventricular dysfunction. Drug toxicity (sympathomimetics, theophylline) is a less common cause(9).

### Therapy:

Therapy should be initially directed at the underlying cause. Correction of hypoxemia and acidosis and careful use of bronchodilator therapy (guided by blood levels when possible) in the patient with chronic obstructive pulmonary disease (COPD) are essential.

Electrical cardioversion is rarely successful in producing sustained sinus rhythm. Digoxin, quinidine, and propranolol have all been reported to be of limited value in either chemical cardioversion or control of the ventricular response rate(6-8). A recent study suggests that intravenous verapamil is a particularly effective agent in controlling the ventricular response rate(10). It should not be used in patients with marginal ventricular function due to its depressant effects on myocardial contractility. In patients with COPD, verapamil will not worsen airway resistance, and its effects upon ventilation/perfusion mismatch (due to pulmonary vascular dilatation) are unlikely to seriously worsen hypoxemia.

## ATRIAL FIBRILLATION

### Description:

Atrial fibrillation is the most common of the supraventricular tachyarrhythmias. It is the result of multiple atrial foci discharging nearly simultaneously. There are no P waves, and effective atrial contraction does not occur. This chaotic electrical activity does produce undulating deflections of varying sizes and shapes on the surface ECG ("f" waves--best seen in V1, II, III, and aVF). Although atrial

electrical impulses are generated at frequencies of 400-700/min, the
number of impulses reaching the ventricles is limited by the refractory
period of the AV node.  In the absence of AV node disease or drugs which
alter the refractory period or conduction velocity of the AV node, 140-180
impulses/min can transverse the AV node at irregular intervals and in a
random fashion.  An irregularly irregular ventricular response rate (QRS
complexes with varying R-R intervals) results.  Atrial fibrillation with
extremely low ventricular response rates (less than 70) reflecting high-
grade AV block may be seen in digitalis toxicity and in patients with sick
sinus syndrome.

Figure 2.6 shows an example of atrial fibrillation in a patient who
was not receiving drugs which affect AV conduction.  P waves are not
evident and irregular undulations ( f  waves) can be seen between R waves.
The R-R interval is irregular and the ventricular response rate is 160/min.

**Figure 2.6 Atrial Fibrillation**

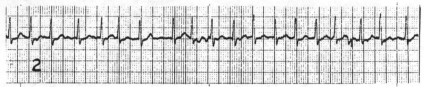

The etiology of atrial fibrillation is thought to be associated with
atrial myocardial tissue injury/damage and elevated atrial pressure(11).
The risk of developing atrial fibrillation has been related to left atrial
dimension as determined by echocardiography.  Similarly, successful
conversion to and maintenance of sinus rhythm appears dependent upon left
atrial size(12,13).  Chronic atrial fibrillation with or without
associated cardiovascular disease has been associated with an increased
mortality rate(14).  Atrial fibrillation complicating acute myocardial
infarction is also associated with an increased death rate(15).

Although atrial fibrillation is the most common cause of an
irregularly irregular rhythm, it must be distinguished from other rhythm
disturbances which may mimic it.

**Table 2.1**
**Irregularly Irregular Rhythm:  Differential Diagnosis**

1.   Atrial flutter with variable AV block
2.   Multifocal atrial tachycardia or chaotic atrial rhythm
3.   Sinus tachycardia with variable AV or SA block
4.   Automatic atrial tachycardia with variable AV block
5.   Marked sinus arrhythmia

Causes:

Population-based data from the Framingham study indicate that atrial fibrillation is most often associated with or caused by coronary heart disease, congestive heart failure, hypertensive cardiovascular disease, and rheumatic heart disease(14). Of note is the fact that 31% of the population developed atrial fibrillation in the absence of clinically identifiable cardiovascular disease.

Other causes include: mitral and aortic valve disease of nonrheumatic origin, hypertrophic cardiomyopathy, and alcohol abuse ("holiday heart syndrome").

**Therapy** (atrial fibrillation with a rapid ventricular response):

**In the hemodynamically unstable patient** (systolic blood pressure of <90 mm Hg, cool clammy skin, altered mentation, and/or chest pain), **urgent electrical synchronized cardioversion is indicated.** If the patient is conscious, sedation with intravenous diazepam (5-10 mg) or a short-acting barbiturate (Brevital; dose titrated to response) should be given prior to cardioversion. Alternatively, morphine sulphate can be given in incremental doses; sedation with morphine has the advantage of being rapidly reversed with the narcotic antagonist naloxone (0.8-1.2 mg). In the synchronized mode, sequential countershocks of 100, 200, 300, and 360 W/sec should be administered as necessary. If the patient is taking digoxin, atrial fibrillation with a rapid irregular ventricular response is not an arrhythmia associated with digitalis toxicity; it is a manifestation of subtherapeutic digoxin concentration. Cardioversion can be safely performed in patients with subtoxic serum digoxin concentrations(16).

If the first attempts at cardioversion are unsuccessful or atrial fibrillation recurs shortly after cardioversion to sinus rhythm, procainamide can be given intravenously at a rate of 30 mg/min to a maximum dose of 20 mg/kg. This regimen has been shown to be efficacious for chemical cardioversion of recent- or new-onset atrial fibrillation in patients without left atrial enlargement(17). If chemical cardioversion is successful, a procainamide constant infusion should be started (2-4 mg/min) and rapid digitalization begun (to control the ventricular response rate if fibrillation recurs). If atrial fibrillation with a rapid ventricular response and hemodynamic compromise persists after procainamide, electrical cardioversion can be attempted again. Procainamide is of value in atrial fibrillation because it decreases atrial automaticity, as well as prolonging the AV node refractory period. The patient should be closely monitored during procainamide administration because the drug may depress myocardial contractility or cause vasodilatation. The drug prolongs the QRS duration as well as the QT interval.

Electrical cardioversion may not be necessary in the patient with clinical evidence of hypoperfusion and atrial fibrillation with a ventricular response rate of <120/min. If the ventricular response rate is irregular and between 80-120/min, other causes of hypoperfusion should be considered (e.g., myocardial infarction and ventricular dysfunction, hypovolemia, pulmonary embolism). If the response rate is <80/min and irregular or regular, digitalis toxicity should be considered if the patient is taking digoxin. Electrical cardioversion in the setting of digitalis toxicity is associated with a high complication rate(18).

**In the hemodynamically stable patient,** cardioversion or rate control are the available options.

**Cardioversion.** Attempted electrical or chemical cardioversion is most likely to be successful (i.e., conversion to and maintenance of sinus rhythm) in patients with recent onset atrial fibrillation, those with a left atrial size of <5 cm, and those with an associated treatable illness (12,13) (e.g., hyperthyroidism, infection, pulmonary embolism, acute respiratory failure). In the stable patient, initial rate control with digoxin and treatment of intercurrent illness, if present, is recommended, followed by echocardiography to assess atrial dimensions.

If left atrial size is <5 cm and the duration of atrial fibrillation is brief (less than 3 days), intravenous loading with procainamide (as described above) followed by electrical cardioversion if needed is often successful. Alternatively, quinidine (300 mg every 4-6 hours for 6-8 doses) can be added to ongoing digoxin therapy. If the addition of quinidine does not produce a chemical conversion, elective electrical cardioversion can be attempted. The risk of an embolic event associated with conversion is low if atrial fibrillation is of brief duration and systemic anticoagulation is not necessary(19).

If left atrial size is <5 cm and the duration of atrial fibrillation more than 3 days, anticoagulation with warfarin (Coumadin) for 3 weeks prior to attempted chemical or electrical cardioversion is recommended. Pharmacologic or electrical cardioversion of prolonged atrial fibrillation is associated with a small risk of systemic embolization (3%), which can be reduced (1%) if anticoagulants are used(20). It is recommended that antithrombotic therapy be continued until sinus rhythm has been maintained for 4 weeks(19).

If left atrial size is >5 cm, the duration of atrial fibrillation is brief, and it is felt that the patient would substantially benefit from resumption of effective atrial contraction, cardioversion can be attempted. However, it is unlikely that sinus rhythm will be maintained for more than a brief period of time (weeks to months).

**Rate Control.** In the hemodynamically stable patient with chronic atrial fibrillation and a left atrial size of >5 cm, chemical or electrical cardioversion is unlikely to be successful(12, 13). In such patients, control of the ventricular response should be the goal of therapy. Digoxin is the drug of choice and can be combined with quinidine, if necessary, for long-term management. Quinidine decreases the renal clearance of digoxin, and combined digoxin/quinidine therapy may produce "toxic" serum concentrations of digoxin(21). Intravenous verapamil (5-10 mg) can also be used for rapid rate control in patients with normal or slightly depressed ventricular function(22). A beta blocker combined with digoxin may be efficacious for chronic therapy in patients without a contraindication to beta blocker therapy and who might benefit from other beta blocker effects, e.g., those with essential hypertension, patients who have had a recent myocardial infarction, and patients with ventricular arrhythmias.

**Anticoagulation** has been recommended for most patients with chronic atrial fibrillation based upon a recent literature review (19). Chronic anticoagulation is not without risks, and its benefits and risks should be assessed for each patient.

Table 2.2
**Long-Term Antithrombotic Therapy in Atrial Fibrillation (Summary of ACCP-NHLBI National Conference on Antithrombotic Therapy)**(19)

1.   It is strongly recommended that chronic long-term warfarin therapy be used in patients with atrial fibrillation who have documented systemic embolism.

2.   It is strongly recommended that long-term warfarin therapy be used in patients with atrial fibrillation and associated mitral valve disease or cardiomyopathy.

3.   In atrial fibrillation associated with other forms of nonvalvular heart disease, data are inconclusive on whether anticoagulant therapy should be used.

4.   It is strongly recommended that warfarin therapy be instituted in patients with atrial fibrillation and thyrotoxicosis and that therapy be continued for 4 weeks after conversion to sinus rhythm and the re-establishment of the euthyroid state.

5.   It is recommended that patients with idiopathic atrial fibrillation without associated heart disease should not receive long-term antithrombotic therapy.


**ATRIAL FLUTTER**

Atrial flutter is a disorder of atrial impulse formation, is less commonly encountered than atrial fibrillation, and most frequently is an unstable rhythm, i.e., spontaneous conversion to sinus rhythm or atrial fibrillation often occurs.  Atrial flutter may be the result of localized atrial re-entry or be of focal, ectopic origin due to enhanced automaticity(23).  Electrical atrial depolarization occurs in an organized manner, and atrial contraction is present.  However, depolarization of the atria is abnormal and often produces diagnostic findings on the surface ECG.

Atrial depolarization occurs at a regular rate, most commonly 280-320/min, and usually is initiated by a re-entry or an ectopic focus in the lower part of the right atrium.  The resulting ECG deflection representing atrial depolarization is most often directed superiorly and leftward, in contrast to the normal inferior and leftward orientation.  During atrial flutter, atrial depolarization produces flutter or "F" waves, which are most easily recognized as regular negative deflections in leads II, III, and aVF.  The absence of an isoelectric period between R waves may result in the typical "saw-toothed" pattern in leads 2, 3, and aVF.

The ventricular rate (frequency and regularity of QRS complexes) during atrial flutter is primarily dependent upon the refractory period/conduction velocity of the AV node.  Atrial flutter is almost always associated with a physiologic AV block.  A physiologic 2:1 AV block occurs most often and results in QRS complexes which occur at a regular rate of 140-160/min.  At this AV response rate, atrial flutter is often misdiagnosed as sinus tachycardia, as the typical saw-tooth pattern in the inferior leads (II, III, aVF) is infrequently present.  The saw-tooth pattern is more often recognized in the inferior leads at higher degrees of AV block (Figure 2.7).  The AV conduction ratio during atrial flutter may be altered by AV node disease, autonomic nervous system variability, or drugs which affect AV node conduction velocity or refractory period (digoxin, type 1A antiarrhythmics).  AV block may be "fixed" (regular R-R interval) or variable (varying R-R interval which is divisible by the inherent atrial rate, e.g., 3:1, 4:1, etc.).  Atrial flutter may infrequently be conducted in 1:1, resulting in a rapid ventricular response.

The clinical and ECG diagnosis of atrial flutter in hemodynamically stable patients without diagnostic ECG findings can be facilitated by physiologic maneuvers which increase the degree of AV block (properly performed carotid sinus massage or Valsalva maneuver).  These clinical interventions often increase the degree of AV block and facilitate recognition of  F  waves.

Figure 2.7A shows an example of atrial flutter recorded in standard lead II. The R-R intervals are regular at a rate of 140/min (2:1 AV block). The rhythm strip in Figure 2.7B was recorded during carotid sinus massage. As the degree of AV block increases (2:1 to 4:1), characteristic saw-tooth F waves of atrial flutter become apparent (rate, 280/min).

**Figure 2.7   Atrial Flutter**

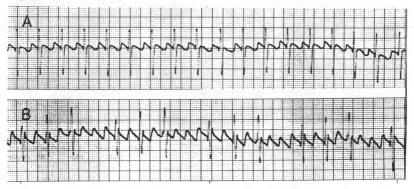

**Causes:**   See Atrial Fibrillation.

**Therapy:**

The management of atrial flutter is similar to that of atrial fibrillation and is dictated by the overall hemodynamic response to the rhythm disturbance.

**In the hemodynamically compromised patient** (systolic blood pressure of <90 mm Hg, cool clammy skin, altered mentation, and/or chest pain) with atrial flutter and a rapid ventricular response rate, **urgent synchronized electrical cardioversion is indicated.** A conscious patient should be sedated (diazepam, Brevital, or morphine). In the synchronized mode, the first shock should be delivered at an energy dose of 50-100 W/sec. Conversion of atrial flutter can usually be accomplished at low energy levels. Countershock most often is followed by one of 3 outcomes:

1.   **Sinus Rhythm.** If clinical signs of hypoperfusion are absent, the patient should be closely monitored. If frequent PACs are noted, therapy with P.O. quinidine, procainamide, or disopyramide can be initiated to decrease atrial automaticity as well as prolong AV conduction time if atrial flutter recurs or atrial fibrillation

develops. If clinical signs of hypoperfusion persist after conversion to sinus rhythm, a fluid challenge with 250-500 ml of normal saline can be administered. If evidence of hypoperfusion persists, invasive hemodynamic monitoring with a flotation pulmonary artery catheter may be required.

2. **Atrial Fibrillation.** Atrial flutter is an unstable cardiac rhythm and often spontaneously "converts" to atrial fibrillation. Countershock of atrial flutter is often followed by atrial fibrillation. It has been our experience that patients who are hemodynamically compromised during atrial flutter at a ventricular response rate of 140-160 are unlikely to improve during atrial fibrillation at a similar ventricular response rate. Clinical signs of hypoperfusion frequently worsen, probably due to the lack of organized atrial contraction during atrial fibrillation. Electrical cardioversion of atrial fibrillation should be attempted as outlined above.

3. **Persistent Atrial Flutter.** Countershock energy dose should be increased at increments of 50 W/sec over the first energy dose until atrial flutter is terminated.

**In the hemodynamically stable patient,** several options are available.

1. **Electrical Cardioversion** (see above). Similar rhythm outcomes should be expected. If pharmacologic therapy (discussed below) is not successful in producing the desired response (rhythm conversion or rate control), electrical cardioversion should be attempted, and the incidence of complications is unlikely to be increased. Electrical cardioversion is the treatment of choice for atrial flutter. Since atrial flutter is most often an unstable or transitional rhythm which produces organized atrial contraction, anticoagulation is not needed prior to definitive treatment(19).

2. **Intravenous Verapamil.** This drug can be safely administered to patients without critical myocardial contractile dysfunction. The ventricular response rate usually decreases due to prolonged AV conduction of supraventricular electrical impulses. Verapamil may convert atrial flutter to sinus rhythm in some instances. A dose of 5-10 mg is usually effective. If hypotension occurs in the previously normotensive patient, 0.5-1.0 gm of calcium chloride should be administered to reverse the peripheral vascular effects of this drug. Intravenous calcium administration has limited effects on the myocardial electrical response to verapamil.

3. **Intravenous Digoxin.** This drug will usually decrease the ventricular response rate but is unlikely to decrease the atrial rate. However, digoxin is a fairly good means to pharmacologically convert atrial flutter to sinus rhythm. It may be of value in

patients with chronic moderate to severe left ventricular dysfunction who are not candidates for intravenous verapamil.

Routine systemic anticoagulation is neither necessary nor recommended in the management of atrial flutter.

## RE-ENTRANT SUPRAVENTRICULAR TACHYARRHYTHMIAS

### AN OVERVIEW

The concept of functional or anatomic dissociation of conduction tissue into two pathways with different conduction velocities and refractory periods is postulated to explain re-entry(24). With dissociation into two pathways, a premature impulse encounters refractoriness (unidirectional block) in one pathway and is conducted slowly in the other. During this period of delayed conduction, the blocked pathway recovers responsiveness. If the two pathways are connected, the impulse can re-enter the previously blocked pathway and be conducted to the chamber of origin in a retrograde fashion. During retrograde conduction, the pathway previously used for antegrade conduction regains responsiveness. Once initiated, impulse conduction over the pathways becomes self-perpetuating. Longitudinal dissociation of conducting tissue into two pathways, one with unidirectional block and the other with prolonged conduction time, is necessary for re-entry to occur. In humans, re-entry has been demonstrated in the SA and AV nodes, atrium, and the His-Purkinje system(25).

Re-entrant tachyarrhythmias can be intentionally induced and terminated in the cardiac electrophysiology lab using an extrastimulus technique and documented with intracardiac recordings. Extrastimuli (paced beats) are delivered at decreasing coupling intervals after a series of sinus beats. A critical coupling interval can be demonstrated and a re-entrant tachycardia induced. Re-entrant tachycardias can also be terminated by an extrastimulus if the delivered impulse enters the "re-entrant loop" and alters the conduction velocity and/or refractoriness of the involved pathways. Electrophysiologic criteria for the diagnosis of a re-entrant tachyarrhythmia include: 1) arrhythmia induction with critically timed extrastimuli; 2) termination of an arrhythmia with an appropriately timed extrastimulus; and 3) arrhythmia induction with sudden cessation of pacing at a defined critical pacing rate(25).

### SUPRAVENTRICULAR TACHYCARDIA (SVT) - AV NODAL RE-ENTRY

The pathways utilized for re-entry lie within the AV node. An episode of SVT is initiated by a closely coupled PAC. The P' wave produced by the premature atrial depolarization is morphologically different from the sinus P wave and the P'R interval of the PAC is usually longer than the PR interval of sinus beats. This is due to the fact that atrial depolarization has occurred prematurely and the AV node has not completely repolarized following the preceding sinus beat. If "longitudinal dissociation" has occurred, a regular tachyarrhythmia will result. The ventricular rate is regular and usually between 160-260/minute. Each impulse is conducted back to the atria, but the sequence of atrial depolarization is abnormal, beginning in the lower portion of the right atrium and proceeding superiorly and leftward. Abnormal atrial depolarization may be recognized by "inverted" P waves in the inferior ECG leads (II, III, aVF). In approximately 30% of patients with SVT and AV nodal reentry, an inverted retrograde P wave will be seen to closely follow each QRS complex. If P waves are seen, they are regular, occur at a rate equal to the ventricular rate (there is no AV block), and the R-P interval is usually less than one-half the R-R interval. However, in most cases (>60%) atrial depolarization occurs during inscription of the QRS complex and a retrograde P wave is not seen(26).

Figure 2.8 demonstrates an episode of SVT due to AV node re-entry. As demonstrated in the ladder diagram, the underlying sinus rhythm is interrupted by PACs which are nonconducted. Ectopic P' waves deform the T wave and are not conducted to the ventricles due to the recovery periods of the conduction system. The third PAC induces a rapid, regular tachyarrhythmia (ventricular rate 160/min) due to AV nodal re-entry. As is typical, retrograde P waves are not seen.

**Figure 2.8 AV Node Re-Entry**

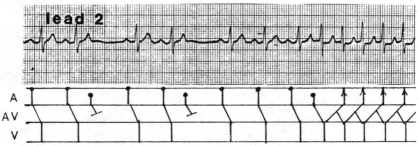

## SVT - RE-ENTRY UTILIZING A CONCEALED BYPASS TRACT (CBT)

This mechanism is similar to that of SVT with AV node re-entry; however, an extranodal conduction pathway is used for retrograde conduction to the atria(27). This extranodal pathway can conduct impulses **only** in a retrograde direction. Patients with Wolff-Parkinson-White (WPW) syndrome also have an extranodal conduction pathway (bypass tract), but it can conduct impulses in both a retrograde or antegrade direction. Antegrade conduction via the extranodal pathway during normal sinus rhythm (NSR) in WPW produces the characteristic "delta wave." Patients with an extranodal conduction pathway capable of only retrograde conduction are said to have a CBT because a delta wave is not inscribed during sinus rhythm.

An episode of SVT is initiated in the same manner as described previously for SVT with AV node re-entry.  The ventricular rate is regular but slightly faster than in SVT with AV node re-entry.  The sequence of atrial depolarization is again abnormal or inverted P waves (leads II, III, and aVF) following each QRS complex, which will be seen in almost all patients(26).  The R-P interval is usually less than one-half of the R-R interval.  During the SVT, a negative P wave is usually seen in lead I in patients with a concealed bypass tract but not in patients with SVT and AV node re-entry(27).  A re-entrant SVT via a CBT is frequently characterized by QRS complexes which vary in amplitude from beat to beat(28).

## SVT WITH SA NODE RE-ENTRY

A PAC usually depolarizes the SA node, resulting in a characteristic noncompensatory pause.  However, an early PAC can encounter block in one portion of the sinus node, enter sinus nodal tissue in another portion, and traverse the nodal tissue slowly enough so that the emerging impulses are able to excite the atria.  Thus, the SA node, in a manner similar to the AV node, can provide pathways for re-entry.  SVT is initiated by a PAC, but subsequent P waves are normal (upright in leads II, III, and aVF) and morphologically similar to sinus beats since the SA node serves as the site of origin(26).  The atrial rate is regular (160-260/min).  AV block (fixed or variable) may occur since the AV node is not a part of the re-entrant loop.  1:1 AV conduction can also occur.  The R-P interval is usually greater than one-half the R-R interval.  Carotid sinus massage (CSM) or a Valsalva maneuver may terminate the rhythm disturbance.

SVT with SA node re-entry is not common and is frequently misdiagnosed because it may mimic sinus tachycardia with AV block and SVT due to an automatic atrial ectopic focus.

## AUTOMATIC ATRIAL TACHYCARDIA

An episode of SVT may also result from the rapid firing of an automatic ectopic focus within the atria.  This rhythm disturbance has been traditionally called "nonparoxysmal atrial tachycardia."  Although it is initiated by a PAC, the coupling interval is not typically short.  The ectopic P' wave vector is usually normal (directed inferiorly and leftward); hence, upright P waves will be noted in leads II, III, and aVF.  P wave morphology will be slightly different from that of sinus beats.  The R-P interval is usually greater than one-half the R-R interal.  AV block may occur; it does not occur in SVT with AV node re-entry or SVT with a CBT.  The ventricular rate may be regular or irregular, depending upon whether the degree of AV block is variable or fixed.  1:1 AV conduction can occur.  Because this rhythm does not involve a re-entry "loop," vagal maneuvers which alter AV conduction (carotid sinus massage, Valsalva maneuver) will not terminate the arrhythmias but may increase the degree of AV block.

An automatic atrial tachycardia is shown in Figure 2.9.  P' waves are shown with arrowheads.  These P' waves are upright in lead 3 (normal atrial depolarization vector) and are regular at a rate of 260/min.  The ventricular rate is also regular at 130/min (2:1 AV block).

**Figure 2.9 Automatic Atrial Tachycardia**

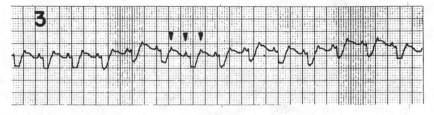

## THE VALUE OF THE ECG IN DEFINING SVT MECHANISM

Careful inspection of the 12-lead ECG during an episode of SVT may be of value in suggesting the underlying electrophysiologic mechanism(29).

**Table 2.3**
**Summary of ECG Findings in SVT**

|  | SVT– AV Node Re-Entry | SVT– CBT | SVT– Automatic Focus or SA Node Re-Entry |
|---|---|---|---|
| Approximate Frequency as a Cause of SVT | 70% | 20% | 10% |
| P Waves in II, III, and aVF | Relatively uncommon | Always | Always |
| P Wave Orientation | Inverted | Inverted | Upright |
| R-P Interval | <1/2 R-R | <1/2 R-R | >1/2 R-R |
| P Wave in Lead I | Upright | Inverted | Upright |
| AV Block | Never | Never | Common |
| Functional Bundle Branch Block | Uncommon | Common | Uncommon |
| Effects of CSM | No change or terminate | No change or terminate | May increase AV block but does not terminate |

## Therapy:

Short runs of these tachyarrhythmias are usually well tolerated and require no specific therapy other than possible PAC suppression to prevent further recurrence. Prolonged episodes may require medical therapy and/or electrical cardioversion. Since these tachyarrhythmias typically result from "re-entry" within the AV node, one must interrupt the critical relation of conduction and refractoriness in the pathways of the AV node.

If the patient is hemodynamically stable, proceed with medical management as outlined below. If the patient is clinically unstable, proceed with sedation (diazepam or Brevital) and synchronized cardioversion utilizing 50 W/sec. Respirations will generally need to be observed carefully and/or assisted during maximum sedation.

## Treatment of Supraventricular Tachycardia of Re-entrant Origin(11):

1. **Carotid Sinus Massage.** Massage either the right or left carotid independently for 10-15 sec while observing a monitor. The arrhythmia will either convert to normal sinus rhythm or will remain unchanged.

2. **Valsalva Maneuver.** Frequently helpful, especially when combined with CSM. Continue CSM after Valsalva maneuver is released.

3. **Verapamil.** Verapamil is currently the only available calcium channel blocking agent in the United States which can be given intravenously and is the drug of choice for termination of acute episodes of AV nodal re-entrant tachycardia. The drug prolongs AV node conduction time via its effects on slow calcium channels. It should be given as a slow IV bolus at a dose of 0.1 mg/kg (5-10 mg). Conversion to sinus rhythm usually occurs within minutes of administration. Verapamil terminates AV nodal re-entrant tachycardia in >90% of patients. The drug is **contraindicated** in patients with moderate to severe LV dysfunction, those taking beta blockers, and patients with a systolic BP of <90 mm Hg during the tachyarrhythmia. IV administration is not uncommonly complicated by hypotension due to the effects of verapamil on peripheral vascular resistance. This side effect can be treated by administering IV calcium chloride (500-1,000 mg). The AV nodal effects of verapamil are not substantially affected by $CaCl_2$.

4. **Digoxin.** IV doses generally of little value in acute therapy due to slow onset of action (usually >2 hours). However, the drug may be given acutely with an eye to using digoxin for long-term therapy.

5. **Atrial pacemaker.** This method frequently will capture the atria and lead to normal sinus rhythm. Set the atrial pacer to a rate faster than the SVT and then abruptly terminate pacing, looking for

resumption of normal sinus rhythm. This method is especially helpful in open-heart surgery patients who may have atrial epicardial wires in place postoperatively.

## ATRIOVENTRICULAR CONDUCTION DEFECTS

A disturbance in impulse conduction from atria to ventricles may occur at the level of the SA node, internodal pathways, AV node, His bundle, bundle branches, or Purkinje network. Although the terms AV block and AV dissociation are often used interchangeably, they are separate entities with markedly differing mechanisms.

AV block may be due to an organic lesion along the conduction pathway, an increase in inherent refractoriness of the conduction pathway, or marked shortening of the supraventricular cycle with encroachment on the normal refractory period. The first two causes are pathologic; the last is physiologic (as exemplified by atrial flutter). AV block may be classified as partial or complete, permanent or temporary, or according to the site of the block (AV nodal or infranodal).

## FIRST DEGREE AV BLOCK (1° AVB)

### Description:

Each supraventricular impulse is conducted to the ventricles, but more slowly than normal. Electrocardiographically, 1° AVB is reflected by a prolonged PR interval (>0.20 sec) that is constant from beat to beat. In the example (Figure 2.10), the PR interval is 0.32 sec. The AV node is usually the site of block, but delay may occur at the level of the internodal pathways, His bundle, or bundle branches (one bundle branch may be completely blocked with delay occurring in the opposite bundle branch). The intensity of the first heart sound tends to decrease as the PR interval becomes longer.

**Figure 2.10**

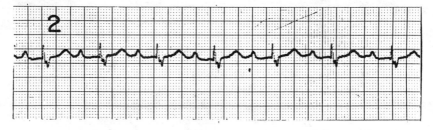

## Causes:

Causes include increased parasympathetic tone, drugs which prolong AV conduction (e.g., digoxin, propranolol), and conduction system disease (e.g., fibrosis, inflammation with myocarditis).

## Therapy:

$1^0$ AVB alone does not produce symptoms and requires no therapy. Digoxin may cause $1^0$ AVB, but this ECG finding is usually not considered a sign of digoxin toxicity unless the PR interval exceeds 0.24 sec.

## SECOND DEGREE AV BLOCK ($2^0$ AVB)

Some supraventricular impulses are conducted to the ventricles while others are blocked. There are two types of $2^0$ AVB and this distinction is prognostically and therapeutically important.

## $2^0$ AVB, Mobitz Type I (Wenckebach)

## Description:

Type I $2^0$ AVB is characterized by progressive prolongation of the PR interval, indicating a progressive decrease in conduction velocity ("decremental conduction") before a P wave is completely blocked (30,31). This form of block almost always occurs at the level of the AV node, but the phenomenon of decremental conduction and "Wenckebach periodicity" has been reported in other conducting tissue (30). Usually only a single impulse is blocked and the cycle is repeated. Longer pauses may be interrupted by escape beats (junctional, ventricular). Repetition of such cycles results in "group beating," e.g., three sinus beats are conducted with progressively increasing PR intervals and the fourth sinus beat is completely blocked and a QRS complex is not inscribed. Such a "group" would be referred to as 4:3 conduction. The conduction ratio is usually constant but it may vary, e.g., 4:3 to 3:2.

In addition to gradual prolongation of the PR interval, typical Wenckebach periodicity is characterized by a decreasing R-R interval prior to the blocked sinus impulse. This is due to the fact that the increment of PR prolongation becomes progressively less with each conducted beat, i.e., while the absolute length of the PR interval increases with each beat, the amount of increase is less with each beat after the second beat of the cycle. The P-P interval is usually constant.

In Figure 2.11, 4:3 Wenckebach periodicity is demonstrated. Relevant intervals are shown in seconds. The atrial rate is regular (constant P-P interval). The PR interval increases from beat to beat. The fourth sinus impulse of the cycle is not conducted to the ventricles. During the Wenckebach cycle, the R-R interval can be seen to decrease prior to the dropped beat, because the increment in the PR interval is decreasing. The increment from 0.28 sec to 0.40 sec is 0.12 sec, while the next increment is only 0.06 sec; the R-R thus decreases by 0.06 sec.

**Figure 2.11 Typical Wenckebach (Mobitz I AVB)**

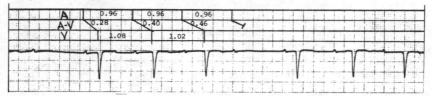

## Atypical Wenckebach

Description:

Rhythms that manifest all the features outlined above represent the typical Wenckebach phenomenon. If many but not all of these features are found, then atypical Wenckebach is said to be present and is due to inconsistent change in the degree of conduction delay from beat to beat. In typical Wenckebach conduction, each impulse is progressively delayed, but with a progressive decrease in the increment of that delay. In atypical Wenckebach, the increment may fail to decrease (PR interval does not change between two consecutive beats), the increment may increase, or a PR interval may be less than the one preceding it. In atypical Wenckebach, conduction delay will tend to increase through the cycle as a whole but will not demonstrate progression from beat to beat. The frequency of atypical Wenckebach conduction increases as the conduction ratio increases--at a conduction ratio greater than 6:5, Wenckebach conduction is almost always atypical(32).

Figure 2.12 demonstrates a Mobitz I AVB with a 9:8 conduction ratio. PR and R-R intervals are included in the ladder diagram. The first four QRS complexes from the right represent the start of the sequence. QRS complexes 2, 3, 4, and 5 from the left represent the end of the cycle. The PR interval does not progressively increase from beat to beat, but over the sequence increases from 0.18 sec to 0.38 sec.

**Figure 2.12 Atypical Wenckebach**

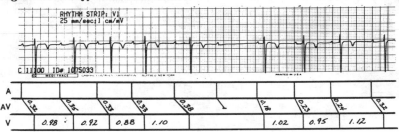

**Causes:**

Causes are the same as for 1° AVB. In addition, this arrhythmia frequently occurs during acute inferior myocardial infarction due to AV nodal ischemia, resulting in increased vagal tone at this level of conduction (in approximately 90% of hearts, the right coronary artery supplies the inferior wall as well as the AV node). This rhythm is a sign of digoxin toxicity in patients taking the medication.

**Therapy:**

**In the hemodynamically stable patient,** acute therapy is not indicated. ICU observation with ECG monitoring is suggested for patients with acute infarction, suspected drug toxicity, or suspected acute myocarditis. In the setting of acute inferior infarction, this arrhythmia is usually transient and well tolerated.

**In the hemodynamically unstable patient,** acute intervention is required. Signs and symptoms of hypoperfusion due to this rhythm disturbance are usually not encountered until the ventricular rate falls below 60/min.

IV atropine should be given in 0.5-mg increments at 5-min intervals until the ventricular response rate increases or a total dose of 2 mg is administered.

Temporary transvenous ventricular pacing should be instituted as soon as possible in patients who do not respond to atropine. Atrial pacing is not likely to be effective since the block is at the level of the

AV node. However, it may be of value in selected cases in which Wenckebach AV conduction is accompanied by profound sinus bradycardia.

If temporary artificial pacing is not immediately available, an isoproterenol infusion (2-20 mu/min) titrated to hemodynamic response can be used with caution. In the setting of acute infarction, the drug may increase myocardial oxygen demand and extend the zone of infarction if demand is not accompanied by an increase in coronary blood flow. In the setting of digoxin toxicity, isoproterenol may worsen ventricular irritability due to its beta-1 effects.

If hypoperfusion persists after an effective ventricular rate increase (>70/min) with atropine or pacing in the setting of acute inferior myocardial infarction, associated right ventricular infarction should be suspected, diagnosed, and appropriate interventions begun (see Chapter 9).

## 2° AVB, Mobitz Type II

### Description:

Block usually occurs below the level of the AV node (infranodal and within the His-Purkinje system)(31). The PR interval is usually normal but may be slightly prolonged. PR intervals do not change measurably from beat to beat, although the PR interval following a blocked impulse may be somewhat shorter. The QRS complexes may be wide (QRS duration, >0.10 sec) since fascicular or bundle branch block (or both) is often present because the infranodal block commonly occurs within the bundle branches. On occasion, QRS complexes of normal duration may be encountered (Figure 2.13). The conduction ratio may be fixed or variable.

Figure 2.13 demonstrates Mobitz Type II second degree block in a three-lead ECG rhythm strip. The PR interval is constant at 0.20 sec until the pause which results from two nonconducted beats. There are three cycles of 3:1 block before 1:1 conduction resumes.

**Figure 2.13 Second Degree AVB, Mobitz Type II**

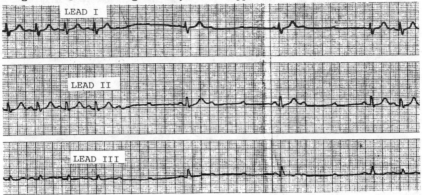

When AV block occurs with a conduction ratio of 2:1, the distinction between Type I or Type II $2^o$ AVB may be difficult since there is no progressive prolongation of the PR interval in 2:1 Type I block. Type I should be suspected if the QRS duration of conducted beats is normal and the presence of more typical Wenckebach periods is noted at other times. 2:1 AVB and wide QRS complexes is most often due to infranodal Type II $2^o$ AVB if the PR interval is normal.

**Causes:**

This arrhythmia is most commonly encountered in chronic degenerative diseases (e.g., Lev's syndrome). It may be seen in acute myocarditis, following cardiac surgery, and in acute anterior myocardial infarction due to distal conduction system ischemia/necrosis.

**Therapy:**

This arrhythmia is usually not a transient phenomenon; it tends to be persistent or recurrent and may progress to complete heart block. It has a more serious prognosis since it is associated with extensive organic damage to the ventricular conduction system. Artificial demand ventricular pacing will be required in most instances. Atropine administration in the acute management is unlikely to be successful but can be attempted as described in Mobitz Type I AVB.

## THIRD DEGREE AV BLOCK ($3^O$ AVB), COMPLETE HEART BLOCK

### Description:

$3^O$ AVB indicates complete absence of atrioventricular conduction. There are two types, which represent a progression in severity from Types I and II $2^O$ AVB.

### $3^O$ AVB at AV Nodal Level

When conduction of supraventricular impulses is blocked completely at the AV node, a "junctional" or AV nodal escape pacemaker initiates ventricular depolarization. This is a stable pacemaker with an inherent firing rate of 40-60/min. Since the escape pacemaker is located above the His bundle, the sequence of ventricular depolarization is normal, resulting in a normal QRS (QRS duration of <0.10 sec). This type of $3^O$ AVB is not uncommon following acute inferior myocardial infarction due to an increase in vagal tone at the level of the AV node. It is usually transient, but may last up to a week.

### Infranodal $3^O$AVB

The ventricles are depolarized by an intrinsic pacemaker located in the bundle branch-Purkinje system. Because the pacemaker lies below the site of the block and the bifurcation of the His bundle, ventricular depolarization does not occur via the normal conducting system and QRS complexes will have a wide configuration (Figure 2.14). A ventricular escape pacemaker has an inherent firing rate of 30-40/min and is relatively unstable, i.e., episodes of ventricular asystole may occur. (Figure 2.4)

Infranodal $3^O$ AVB is indicative of extensive conduction system disease and is often a complication of acute anterior myocardial infarction.

In both types of $3^O$ AVB, atrial and ventricular depolarization are independent, the PR intervals vary in a random fashion, and the atrial rate is faster than the ventricular rate. The ventricular rate is regular. The atrial rate is usually regular but may show sinus arrhythmia (ventriculophasic sinus arrhythmia: P-P intervals that bracket a QRS are shorter than those that do not). Critical differentiating features are QRS morphology and escape pacemaker rate.

Figure 2.14 Infranodal 3° AVB

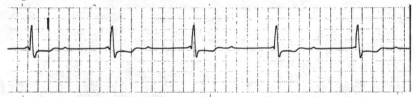

Therapy:

1.   3° AVB at AV Node Level
     Same as for 2° AVB, Mobitz Type I.

2.   Infranodal 3° AVB

     An artificial demand pacemaker will almost always be required.
     Acutely, IV atropine or isoproterenol can be given, but neither
     is likely to be of value in the hemodynamically compromised
     patient.

## ATRIOVENTRICULAR DISSOCIATION (AVD)

Description:

     Atrioventricular dissociation is never a primary diagnosis; it is
always secondary to some other rhythm disturbance.   In AVD the atria and
ventricles are depolarized by separate pacemakers. The atria are
activated by the sinus node.   The ventricles are depolarized by a lower-
level pacemaker at the level of the AV node or within the ventricular
conduction system.   The ventricular rate is either equal to the atrial
rate (isorhythmic AVD) or greater than the atrial rate.   In AV block, the
atrial rate is faster than the ventricular rate.   The lower pacemaker
depolarizes the ventricles because it encounters a nonrefractory
myocardium.   Atrioventricular dissociation may be passive or active.

**Passive AVD**

     When the sinus node fails to depolarize within approximately 1 sec, a
junctional or ventricular escape beat or rhythm may emerge.   If a sinus
impulse should reach the AV junction between escape beats when the AV node
is not refractory, the sinus beat will be conducted to the ventricles.
Therefore, AV block is not present.

Figure 2.15 demonstrates the passive type of AV dissociation.   The first two sinus beats are conducted normally to the ventricles.   A long pause follows the second QRS due to sinus arrest.   The pause is interrupted by a fusion beat and then an accelerated idioventricular rhythm.   Sinus rhythm resumes at the end of the strip.

**Figure 2.15 Passive AVD**

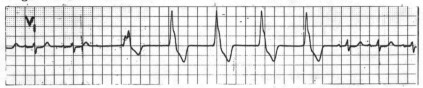

## Active AVD

The discharge rate of the lower pacemaker exceeds or usurps that of the sinus node in the absence of bradycardia.   Hence, it is due to an accelerated junctional or idioventricular rhythm or ventricular tachycardia.

**Therapy:**

In the asymptomatic patient, therapy is often unnecessary.   Therapy should be directed at the underlying cause—the primary rhythm. Atropine may be effective in increasing the sinus rate in passive AVD. Suppressing an accelerated idioventricular rhythm in the presence of a slow sinus rhythm may be deleterious.

## VENTRICULAR ARRHYTHMIAS

### VENTRICULAR EXTRASYSTOLE (PREMATURE VENTRICULAR CONTRACTION)

**Description:**

A premature ventricular contraction (PVC) is a premature impulse of ventricular origin occurring before the next expected sinus beat.   It may arise from a ventricular focus with enhanced automaticity or may represent a form of re-entry within the His-Purkinje system.   Both mechanisms may be operative under different circumstances.   PVCs may be unifocal (identical or nearly identical QRS morphology with a fixed coupling interval) (Figure 2.16) or multifocal (varying QRS morphology and coupling intervals).

Since a PVC originates in the ventricle, ventricular depolarization and repolarization are abnormal, resulting in a wide QRS complex (>0.12

sec) and an ST segment and T wave directed opposite the QRS complex. The SA node is anatomically and "electrically" separated from the ventricles, and a PVC usually does not depolarize the SA node due to refractoriness to retrograde conduction in the AV node. Therefore, the rhythm of the SA node is not disturbed and there is usually a fully compensatory pause. On occasion, the SA node may be depolarized, and a noncompensatory pause will result. In the presence of a slow sinus rhythm, a PVC may occur between two sinus beats, resulting in an "interpolated" PVC (the P-P interval remains unchanged because there is no pause). The sinus impulse following an interpolated PVC usually has a prolonged PR interval, since the AV node is still refractory from incomplete penetration (concealed conduction) by the PVC.

The third and seventh QRS complexes in Figure 2.16 are PVCs of unifocal origin (same morphology and coupling interval) followed by a fully compensatory pause (R-R interval of sinus beats bracketing a PVC is twice that of the basic sinus rate).

**Figure 2.16 Unifocal PVCs**

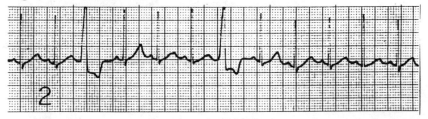

**Causes:**

Causes include acute and chronic myocardial ischemia, cardiomyopathy, electrolyte disturbances (hypokalemia), and drug toxicity (sympathomimetics, digoxin).

**Therapy:**

In the acutely ill patient with an acute myocardial infarction, suspected infarction, acute respiratory failure, following cardiac surgery, etc., lidocaine, given as an IV bolus followed by continuous IV infusion, should be administered (see Chapter 9). Indications for therapeutic intervention in the management of "chronic" PVCs are discussed in Chapter 15.

## VENTRICULAR ESCAPE BEATS (IDIOVENTRICULAR RHYTHM)

### Description:

A ventricular escape beat is an impulse originating from a pacemaker within the His-Purkinje network. It occurs after the next expected supraventricular impulse has failed to occur or be conducted to the ventricles. Such a pacemaker has an intrinsic rate of 30-40/min, and the interval preceding the escape beat is usually greater than 1.5 sec. If more than one escape beat occurs in succession, a ventricular escape (or idioventricular) rhythm and atrioventricular dissociation are present. If the rate is greater than 40/min but less than 100/min, an accelerated idioventricular rhythm (AIVR) is said to be present (Figure 2.17). Escape beats and rhythms have wide QRS complexes, abnormal ST segments, and secondary T waves changes as seen in PVCs.

Figure 2.17 demonstrates AIVR on the top strip which is interrupted by a PVC. The last beat on the top strip is the beginning of a 3-beat interlude of sinus bradycardia which is, in turn, interrupted by the resumption of AIVR when the sinus rate becomes slower than the AIVR rate. The rhythm disturbance is similar to that shown in Figure 2.15.

**Figure 2.17 Accelerated Idioventricular Rhythm**

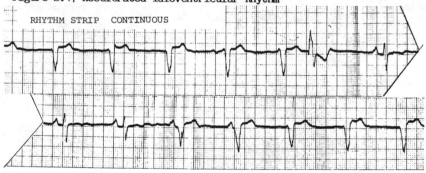

RHYTHM STRIP   CONTINUOUS

### Therapy:

Ventricular escape beats and accelerated idioventricular rhythms are not uncommon following acute myocardial infarction. Suppressant drugs such as lidocaine should not be used in the event that they may represent the only reliable pacemaker. IV atropine sulfate given in 0.5-mg increments every 5 min (total dose, 2 mg) may accelerate the SA node or allow the atria to "capture" the ventricles. Artificial pacing may be required if the dominant rhythm is too slow for adequate perfusion.

# VENTRICULAR PARASYSTOLE

## Description:

Ventricular parasystole refers to the presence of concurrent impulse formation by two pacemakers, one in the SA node and the other in the ventricle. Independent pacemakers may also be noted during AVD, but differences exist between AVD and parasystole. The ventricular parasystolic pacemaker has three important properties not shared by a lower pacemaker in AVD:

1. **Entrance Block.** An electrical impulse cannot enter the parasystolic focus and depolarize it; hence, the parasystolic pacemaker fires at a fixed rate and is not reset by ventricular depolarization.

2. **Intermittent Exit Block.** Despite the fact that impulses are repetitively generated by the parasystolic pacemaker, impulse conduction to the surrounding myocardium does not always occur.

3. **Constant Rate of Discharge.** The constant rate of discharge is evidenced by the fact that the interval between parasystolic beats (interectopic interval) remains constant, or is a multiple of a basic interval. Each impulse may not produce a QRS complex due to existing block or refractoriness of the myocardium from a preceding depolarization.

Parasystolic beats are ventricular ectopic beats with constant QRS morphology, but the coupling interval is usually variable. "Fusion beats" may be seen if the sinus beat reaches the ventricle at approximately the same time that the parasystolic focus discharges.

In the following example of ventricular parasystole (Figure 2.18), the interectopic interval is nearly constant (varies by less than 2%). The first ectopic beat immediately follows the P wave and there is no fusion. The subsequent three ectopic beats demonstrate fusion with progressively more influence from the conducted beat--the QRS complex narrows and the T wave amplitude declines--because the ectopic beat is occurring progressively later after the P wave.

**Figure 2.18**

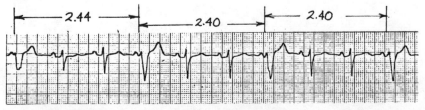

Therapy:

Ventricular parasystole frequently occurs in the presence of severe underlying heart disease. Suppressive drugs (lidocaine) are less effective than in fixed-coupled PVCs. Parasystole can lead to ventricular tachycardia or fibrillation, particularly in the setting of myocardial ischemia or infarction. In the absence of ischemia, the rhythm can be stable for many years.

## VENTRICULAR TACHYCARDIA (VT)

Description:

VT is a ventricular arrhythmia due to reentry within the His-Purkinje network(33). PVCs usually presage its occurrence (see Chapter 15, Sudden Cardiac Death). An episode of VT is constituted by at least three successive ventricular ectopic beats at a rate in excess of 100/min (usual rate, 140-220/min). Because the sequence of ventricular depolarization and repolarization is abnormal, QRS complexes during VT are wide, and distinct ST segments and T waves may not be evident. The basic sinus rhythm may remain intact, leading to antegrade atrial depolarization with AV dissociation. On occasion, the sinus node may "capture" the ventricle (capture beat) or cause fusion beats if the AV node and ventricular myocardium are not refractory. VT is usually a regular rhythm except when a capture beat occurs. Conduction from the ventricle to the atria may occur, resulting in retrograde atrial depolarization. Hence, AV dissociation is not necessary for the diagnosis of VT. Capture and fusion beats will not occur during ventriculo-atrial conduction.

In Figure 2.19 simultaneous V5 and V1 equivalent leads from a Holter monitor recording reveal a single PVC followed by a four-beat burst of VT. The P waves are marked by vertical lines. There is AV dissociation with a constant atrial rate of 94 during the VT which occurs at a rate of 165. The P waves are too close to the ectopic ventricular beats to cause fusion beats.

Figure 2.19 Ventricular Tachycardia

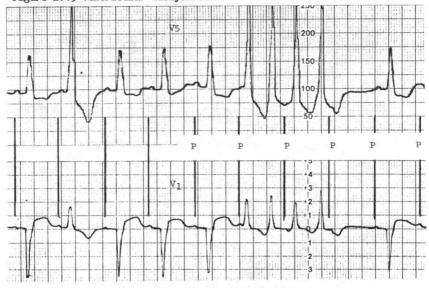

## Causes:

Causes are similar to causes of PVCs.

## Therapy:

If the patient is hemodynamically stable, a lidocaine bolus may be given and a constant infusion of lidocaine initiated. If the patient has clinical signs of hypoperfusion or is in cardiopulmonary arrest, countershock should be administered immediately and CPR initiated (see Chapter 16).

## VENTRICULAR ECTOPY VERSUS ABERRANT VENTRICULAR CONDUCTION

Premature, morphologically bizarre QRS complexes may result from discharge of a ventricular ectopic focus (PVC) or from abnormal or "aberrant" ventricular conduction of a supraventricular impulse. Aberrant ventricular conduction (AVC) occurs when a premature impulse encounters partially refractory ventricular conduction tissue, usually the right bundle branch. The right bundle branch has a longer refractory period than the left bundle branch. The more premature the supraventricular impulse, the more likely that AVC will occur. Because of the disparity in refractory periods of the bundle branches, AVC usually takes the form of a right bundle branch block pattern. Left bundle branch aberration may also occur but is infrequent(34).

The length of the refractory period of the bundle branches is determined by the preceding R-R interval--the refractory period is longer with slow heart rates (long R-R interval) and shorter with fast rates (short R-R interval). A long R-R interval preceding a PAC will facilitate AVC.

Close inspection of the ECG may allow differentiation of a PVC from AVC of a supraventricular impulse, usually a PAC(34).

**The following ECG features are suggestive of a PAC with AVC** (Figure 2.20):

- An rSR' pattern in lead V1.
- A premature P' wave preceding the bizarre QRS complex. The P wave morphology may be different from that of sinus P waves and the PR interval of the PAC is usually longer than that of the normally conducted sinus beats. The premature P wave may be "hidden" in the preceding T wave.
- A noncompensatory pause follows the bizarre QRS complex.
- A QRS duration of $\leq$0.12 sec.
- In atrial fibrillation or in MAT, aberrantly conducted beats resembling PVCs may be seen when short R-R intervals follow long R-R intervals ("long-short cycle sequence"). These beats are often called Ashman beats in recognition of their characterization by Gouaux and Ashman in 1947.

In Figure 2.20 (lead V1), wide QRS complexes are seen to interrupt sinus rhythm. These complexes are triphasic (rSR' or RBBB morphology), and the QRS duration is <0.12 sec. Premature P waves (arrows) can be recognized on the downslope of the preceding T wave, and the PR intervals of the PACs are greater than those of normally conducted sinus beats. The wide QRS complexes are, therefore, the result of aberrant conduction of PACs. Note that the second PAC is less premature than the first and third, and there is no aberrancy.

**Figure 2.20 PACs with Aberrant Ventricular Conduction**

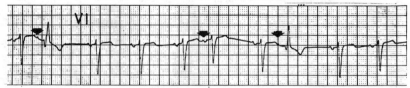

**The following ECG features are suggestive of a PVC** (Figure 2.21):

- A monophasic or biphasic QRS complex in lead V1.
- If the QRS complex is notched ("rabbit ear" pattern), the amplitude of the R wave is greater than that of the R' wave in V1.  If R' wave amplitude is greater than that of the R wave, a PVC may not be confidently distinguished from a PAC with AVC.
- A QS wave in V6.
- A P wave does not precede the bizarre QRS complex.
- QRS duration of >0.16 sec.
- Bizarre QRS complex followed by a fully compensatory pause.

Two PVCs are shown in Figure 2.21 (the second and fourth QRS complexes).  These complexes have a QRS duration of 0.14 sec, are biphasic, and have a rabbit ear pattern (notch on QRS downstroke).  Each is followed by a fully compensatory pause.

**Figure 2.21 Ventricular Ectopy**

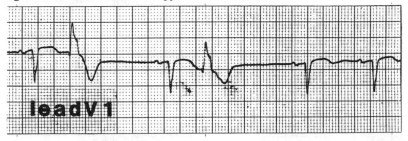

Similar criteria have been reported to aid in the differentiation of sustained ventricular tachycardia (VT) from a sustained supraventricular tachyarrhythmia with aberrant ventricular conduction (SVT-AVC).  These are summarized in Table 2.4(35).

**Table 2.4**
**SVT with Aberration Versus Ventricular Tachycardia**

|  | SVT-AVC | VT |
|---|---|---|
| QRS morphology in V1 | Triphasic (rSR') | Mono- or biphasic |
| R/S ratio in V6 | >1.0 | <1.0 |
| Frontal plane QRS axis | Normal or rightward | <-30° |
| QRS duration | ≤0.14 sec | >0.14 sec |
| Ventricular rate | >170/min | <170/min |
| Fusion beats | No | Yes |
| AV dissociation/V-A conduction | No | Yes |

Careful inspection of the 12-lead ECG with the above differences in mind will most often lead to a correct diagnosis. In more difficult cases, the physical examination may be of help. The presence of AV dissociation during VT may produce "cannon a" waves in the jugular venous pulse pattern and a first heart sound of varying intensity(35). The presence or absence of hypotension is of no differential diagnostic value(36).

In the hemodynamically unstable patient, cardioversion is the treatment of choice, regardless of the origin of the rhythm. In the stable patient, without classic ECG findings for VT or SVT with aberrant conduction, intravenous procainamide (10-12 mg/kg over 30 min) should be administered. Procainamide will not only slow or terminate VT, but can also interrupt a supraventricular tachycardia due to re-entry(37).

Figure 2.22 is an example of ventricular tachycardia (subsequently confirmed with intracardiac recordings). The 12-lead recording meets the criteria for VT as noted in column 2 of Table 2.4.

**Figure 2.22 Ventricular Tachycardia (12-lead ECG)**

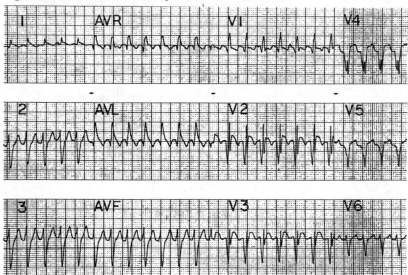

## TORSADES DE POINTES

Description:

The term "torsades de pointes" (twisting of the points) was chosen by Dessertenne in 1966 to describe a new ventricular arrhythmia with unusual characteristics. As initially described, the limb leads show cycles of alternating QRS polarity such that the peaks of the QRS complexes appear to be twisting around the isoelectric line of the recording. In each cycle, the amplitude of consecutive ventricular complexes increases and decreases in a sinusoidal fashion. However, these sinusoidal cycles make up only a portion of the arrhythmia. At other times, the rhythm is that of typical ventricular tachycardia (uniform morphology and polarity of wide ventricular complexes in the monitor lead) (Figure 2.23). This rhythm is also characterized by frequent spontaneous conversion and recurrence(38). If spontaneous conversion occurs, it usually does so within 30 sec of onset of the arrhythmia. Electrical cardioversion may be required to terminate the arrhythmia. **Current opinion is that torsades de pointes should be diagnosed only if the above morphologically distinct ECG pattern is associated with a prolonged correct QT interval between occurrences**(38, 39). In most instances, the corrected QT interval will be >0.60 sec. In the absence of QT prolongation, a diagnosis of polymorphous or atypical ventricular tachycardia is suggested. This distinction is extremely important for acute and chronic management of this unusual ventricular arrhythmia.

The majority of data indicates that torsades de pointes is a re-entrant ventricular tachyarrhythmia due to increased temporal dispersion of myocardial recovery times (repolarization rates)(38). The arrhythmia is usually precipitated by a ventricular premature beat occurring in late diastole and usually falling on the summit of a prolonged T-U wave.

**Figure 2.23 Torsades de Pointes**

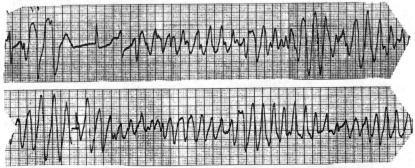

## Causes:

Causes include 1) congenital QT prolongation syndromes; 2) drug-induced acquired QT prolongation (class IA antiarrhythmics [quinidine, disopyramide, procainamide], phenothiazines, tricyclic antidepressants); 3) complete heart block; 4) hypokalemia; 5) hypomagnesemia; 6) intrinsic heart disease (ischemic heart disease, myocarditis); 7) CNS disease; 8) liquid protein diets.

## Therapy:

A correct diagnosis is critical in acute and chronic management. Use of class IA antiarrhythmics for this rhythm disturbance may adversely affect outcome. Treatment aims are to remove or correct the predisposing cause when possible (e.g., stop drugs, correct electrolyte disturbances) and to suppress the arrhythmia until either the QT interval decreases or a diagnosis of congenital QT prolongation is confirmed.

Cardioversion should be used for prolonged episodes. However, because this arrhythmia tends to recur, the therapeutic objective should be to prevent recurrence(38, 40).

**Intravenous magnesium sulphate** (effective dose, approximately 2 gm) has recently been shown to be of value in preventing recurrence, even in patients with normal serum magnesium levels. Its mechanism of effect has not been conclusively established. Since this drug has not produced adverse effects and can be rapidly administered in the acute setting, magnesium may be the drug of first choice for management of this arrhythmia.

**An isoproterenol infusion** (2-10 mu/min) can be used for acute control. Isoproterenol reduces the dispersion of myocardial recovery by a direct effect and indirectly by increasing the sinus node discharge rate. The QT interval decreases with increasing heart rate. However, this drug increases myocardial oxygen demand and decreases peripheral vascular resistance. It should be used with caution, especially in patients with intrinsic heart disease.

**Temporary overdrive pacing** has been particularly successful in preventing recurrence. If AV conduction is intact, atrial pacing is the preferred technique. Most agree that overdrive pacing is the definitive method for preventing recurrence.

**Temporary blockade of the left stellate ganglion by injection of lidocaine** may also be effective. However, this intervention requires skill and is only a temporary measure.

**Bretylium** (5 mg/kg) has also been successfully used in a limited study population.

The class IA antiarrhythmics should not be used since they will further increase the QT interval. Lidocaine produces inconsistent results.

In patients with acquired QT prolongation, overdrive pacing can be discontinued when the predisposing cause has been corrected and the QT interval has returned to normal. Prophylactic drug therapy is not needed.

In patients subsequently diagnosed as having congenital QT prolongation, long-term treatment with oral propranolol has been shown to be effective in symptomatic patients. Surgical sympathectomy has been recommended for those symptomatic patients who do not respond to propranolol.

## VENTRICULAR FIBRILLATION

### Description:

This is a chaotic ventricular rhythm (Figure 2.24) felt to be due to multiple re-entrant foci within the ventricle. Organized electrical activity is not present and since the ventricle does not depolarize as a unit, no ventricular contraction occurs.

### Figure 2.24

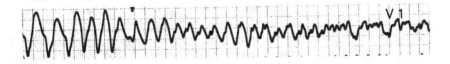

### Therapy:

See Chapter 16, Cardiopulmonary Resuscitation.

# REFERENCES

1.  Standards and guidelines for cardiopulmonary resuscitation and emergency cardiac care. JAMA 255:2948, 1986.

2.  Chadda KD, Lichstein E, Gupta PK, et al.: Effects of atropine in patients with bradyarrhythmia complicating myocardial infarction. Usefulness of an optimum dose for overdrive. Am J Med 63:503, 1977.

3.  Talano JV, Euler D, Randall WC, et al.: Sinus node dysfunction. An overview with emphasis on autonomic and pharmacologic consideration. Am J Med 64:773, 1978.

4.  Weinstein RS: Recognition and management of poisoning with beta-adrenergic blocking agents. Ann Emerg Med 13:1123, 1984.

5.  Singh BN: Intravenous calcium and verapamil--when the combination may be indicated. Int J Cardiol 4:281, 1983 (editorial).

6.  Lipson MJ, Naimi S: Multifocal atrial tachycardia (chaotic atrial tachycardia). Circulation 42:397, 1970.

7.  Wang K, Goldfarb BL, Gobel FL, et al.: Multifocal atrial tachycardia. A clinical analysis in 41 cases. Arch Intern Med 137: 161, 1977.

8.  Shine KI, Kastor JA, Yurchak PM: Multifocal atrial tachycardia. Clinical and electrocardiographic features in 32 patients. N Engl J Med 279:344, 1968.

9.  Marchlinski FE, Miller JM: Atrial arrhythmias exacerbated by theophylline. Response to verapamil and evidence for triggered activity in man. Chest 88:931, 1985.

10. Levine JH, Michael JR, Guarnieri T: Treatment of multifocal atrial tachycardia with verapamil. N Engl J Med 312:21, 1985.

11. Keefe DL, Miura D, Somberg JC: Supraventricular tachyarrhythmias: Their evaluation and therapy. Am Heart J 111:1150, 1986.

12. Henry WL, Morganroth J, Pearlman AS, et al.: Relation between echocardiographically determined left atrial size and atrial fibrillation. Circulation 53:273, 1976.

13. Mancini GBJ, Golderberger AL: Cardioversion of atrial fibrillation: Consideration of embolization, anticoagulation, prophylactic pacemaker, and long-term success. Am Heart J 104:617, 1982.

14. Kannel WB, Abbott RD, Savage DD, et al.: Epidemiologic features of chronic atrial fibrillation: The Framingham Study. N Engl J Med 306:1018, 1982.

15. DeSanctis RW, Block P, Hutter AM: Tachyarrhythmias in myocardial infarction. Circulation 45:681, 1982.

16. Mann DL, Maisel AS, Atwood JE, et al.: Absence of cardioversion-induced ventricular arrhythmias in patients with therapeutic digoxin levels. J Am Coll Cardiol 5:883, 1985.

17. Halpern SW, Ellrodt G, Singh BN, et al.: Efficacy of intravenous procainamide infusion in converting atrial fibrillation to sinus rhythm: Relation to left atrial size. Br Heart J 44:589, 1980.

18. Lown B: Cardioversion and the digitalized patient. J Am Coll Cardiol 5:889, 1985.

19. Dunn M, Alexander J, de Silva R, et al.: Antithrombotic therapy in atrial fibrillation. Chest 89 (suppl):68S, 1986.

20. Bjerkelund CJ, Orning OM: The efficacy of anticoagulant therapy in preventing embolism related to D. C. electrical cardioversion of atrial fibrillation. Am J Cardiol 23:208, 1969.

21. Doering W: Quinidine-digoxin interaction. Pharmacokinetics, underlying mechanism, and clinical implications. N Engl J Med 301:400, 1979.

22. Tammaso C, McDonough T, Parker M, et al.: Atrial fibrillation and flutter. Immediate control and conversion with intravenously administered verapamil. Arch Intern Med 143:877, 1983.

23. Waldo AL, Henthorn RW, Plumb VJ: Atrial flutter--recent observations in man. In Josephson ME, Wellens HJJ (eds): Tachycardias: Mechanisms, Diagnosis, and Treatment. Philadelphia, Lea and Febiger, 1984, pp. 113-135.

24. Josephson ME, Kastor JA: Supraventricular tachycardia: Mechanisms and management. Ann Intern Med 87:346, 1977.

25. Wu D, Denes P: Mechanisms of paroxysmal supraventricular tachycardia. Arch Intern Med 135:437, 1975.

26. Wu D, Denes P, Amat-Y-Leon F, et al.: Clinical, electrocardiographic and electrophysiologic observations in patients with paroxysmal supraventricular tachycardia. Am J Cardiol 42:1045, 1978.

27.  Farshidi A, Josephson ME, Horowitz LN: Electrophysiologic characteristics of concealed bypass tracts: Clinical and electrocardiographic correlates. Am J Cardiol 41:1052, 1978.

28.  Green M, Heddle B, Dassen W, et al.: Value of QRS alternation in determining the site of origin of narrow QRS supraventricular tachycardia. Circulation 68:368, 1983.

29.  Josephson ME: Paroxysmal supraventricular tachycardia: An electrophysiologic approach. Am J Cardiol 41:1123, 1978.

30.  Cabeen WR, Roberts NK, Child JS: Recognition of the Wenckebach phenomenon. West J Med 129:521, 1978.

31.  Kastor JA: Atrioventricular block (Part I). N Engl J Med 292:462, 1975. Atrioventricular block (Part II). N Engl J Med 292:572, 1975.

32.  Denes P, Levy L, Pich A, et al.: The incidence of typical and atypical A-V Wenckebach periodicity. Am Heart J 89:26, 1975.

33.  Josephson ME, Horowitz LN, Farshidi A, et al.: Recurrent sustained ventricular tachycardia. 1. Mechanisms. Circulation 57:431, 1978.

34.  Marriott HJL, Conover MHB: Advanced Concepts in Arrhythmias. St. Louis, The Mosby Company, St. Louis, 1983, pp. 244-267.

35.  Wellens HJJ, Bar FWHM, Lie KI: The value of the electrocardiogram in the differential diagnosis of a tachycardia with a widened QRS complex. Am J Med 64:27, 1978.

36.  Morady F, Baerman JM, DiCarlo LA Jr, et al.: A prevalent misconception regarding wide-complex tachycardias. JAMA 254:2790, 1985.

37.  Wellens HJJ: The wide QRS tachycardia. Ann Intern Med 104:879, 1986 (editorial).

38.  Smith WM, Gallagher JJ: Les torsades de pointes: An unusual ventricular arrhythmia. Ann Intern Med 93:578, 1980.

39.  Tzivoni D, Keren A, Stern S: Torsades de pointes versus polymorphous ventricular tachycardia. Am J Cardiol 52:639, 1983.

40.  Stern S, Keren A, Tzivoni D: Torsades de pointes: Definitions, causative factors, and therapy-experience with sixteen patients. Ann N Y Acad Sci 427:234, 1984.

# Chapter 3

# Exercise Stress Testing

Exercise Stress Testing (EST) is a sensitive and informative examination of the cardiovascular response to exercise. EST is particularly useful in the detection and quantitation of ischemic heart disease (IHD) in those patients at increased risk for its occurrence. For the purposes of this discussion, IHD is used to represent impairment of coronary perfusion usually due to, but not limited to, atherosclerotic coronary artery disease (CAD).

## EXERCISE PHYSIOLOGY

1. The heart extracts 70% of the oxygen carried by each unit of blood perfusing the myocardium and **myocardial metabolism is nearly entirely aerobic.** Therefore, an increase in myocardial oxygen demand during exercise must be matched by an increase in coronary blood flow (supply)or ischemia will result.

2. **Major factors affecting myocardial oxygen demand:**

   - Heart rate (HR)

   - Contractility

   - Wall tension (directly proportional to ventricular pressure x radius)

3. The **"double product" (blood pressure x HR)** shows a good correlation with measured myocardial oxygen consumption during dynamic exercise. Angina occurs at a remarkably constant double product in a given patient with IHD often independent of duration, intensity, or type of exercise performed. In practice, EST is designed to produce an increase in HR of known magnitude, defined as a percentage of the maximal predicted HR of a normal population of matched age and sex (Table 3.1).

Table 3.1
Expected HR Response to Graded Exercise

| Age | Mild | Mod. | Mod.Sev. | Near Max. | Max. |
|-----|------|------|----------|-----------|------|
| 20-29 | 115 | 135 | 155 | 175 | 195 |
| 30-39 | 110 | 130 | 150 | 170 | 190 |
| 40-49 | 106 | 126 | 146 | 166 | 186 |
| 50-59 | 102 | 122 | 142 | 162 | 182 |
| 60+ | 98 | 118 | 138 | 158 | 178 |

4.  In the presence of IHD, coronary blood flow cannot increase
    adequately to meet the demands of the myocardium for oxygen,
    resulting in ischemia and manifested by 1) pain (angina), 2) ECG ST
    segment changes, 3) ventricular dysfunction, 4) arrhythmias, or 5) a
    combination of the above.

5.  Types of exercise:

    - Static:   Isometric sustained muscular contraction against a fixed
                resistance; for example, a handgrip.

    - Dynamic: Rhythmic contractions of extensor and flexor muscle
                groups; for example, a bicycle or treadmill exercise.

    - Combination of static and dynamic exercise.

6.  Why is dynamic exercise preferred in EST?

    - Isometric exercise can produce exaggerated BP response which may
      be detrimental to patients with high blood pressure or CAD.

    - HR response is variable in isometric exercise while it will
      reliably increase during dynamic exercise.

    - Angina pectoris is less reliably provoked during
      isometric exercise.

    - Isometric exercise frequently provokes ventricular
      arrhythmias.

    - ECG changes during isometric exercise may be subtle and obscured by
      muscle tremor artifact.

### WHAT ARE THE INDICATIONS FOR EST?

1.  Differential diagnosis of chest pain; i.e., evaluation of patients
    with symptoms suggestive of IHD.

2.  **Assessment of the level of exercise** at which ischemic manifestations occur in a patient with known IHD.

3.  **Evaluation of therapy** for arrhythmias and angina.

4.  **Evaluation of functional disability** secondary to organic heart disease, e.g., valvular heart disease.

5.  **Evaluation of the asymptomatic patient** over 40 who has multiple risk factors for IHD.

## CONTRAINDICATIONS TO EST

1.  Recent acute myocardial infarction (MI) (4 to 6 weeks), except for submaximal (65% of predicted maximum HR)or symptom-limited EST prior to hospital discharge.

2.  Angina at rest.

3.  Rapid ventricular or atrial arrhythmias.

4.  Advanced atrioventricular (AV) block (unless chronic).

5.  Uncompensated congestive heart failure.

6.  Acute noncardiac illnesses.

7.  Severe aortic stenosis.

8.  BP greater than 170/100 prior to the onset of exercise.

## HOW SAFE IS EST?

In a 73 center study of EST, **mortality** was 0.01%, **morbidity** (arrhythmias and/or prolonged chest pain requiring hospitalization) was 0.04%(1). **Therefore, EST is a safe procedure when done under proper supervision and with the necessary safeguards and equipment.** These include:

1.  Physician's knowledge of the patient's history and physical findings prior to the EST.

2.  Physician present for the entire test.

3.  Continuous monitoring of HR and rhythm, and frequent BP determinations during the procedure and for 10 min thereafter.

4. Emergency equipment readily available, including a defibrillator, airway management equipment, and emergency drugs.

5. Termination of the EST at the appropriate time (see below).

## WHEN TO TERMINATE THE EST

1. Achievement of predicted HR (see Table 3.1).

2. Patient unable to continue due to symptoms of excessive fatigue, claudication, and/or dyspnea.

3. Premature ventricular contractions (PVCs) increasing in frequency and/or ventricular tachycardia.

4. Onset of advanced AV block.

5. Severe angina occurs.

6. Diagnostic ST segment changes clearly obtained on ECG.

7. BP criteria:  systolic greater than 220; diastolic greater than 120 during exercise; or during exercise BP drops to a level below baseline (may indicate left ventricular [LV] dysfunction).

8. Onset of bundle branch block.

9. Failure of the ECG monitoring system.

## EST RECOVERY

Following the termination of the EST, the patient should be observed in a supine position for 10 min with continuous ECG monitoring.  Obtain BP frequently and look for ECG ST segment changes and arrhythmias which commonly occur postexercise.  The ECG should return to baseline prior to releasing the   patient.

## HOW IS THE EST DONE?

1. **Protocols are used which utilize dynamic exercise on a treadmill up to a predicted maximal heart rate for age.** There are many multistage protocols which utilize increments in treadmill elevation and speed; each protocol has its advantages, depending on the patient being tested.  Small increments in workloads of short duration (Ellestad [2] may be better tolerated than larger workloads of longer duration (Bruce [3]), especially in older patients in poor physical condition.  In order to obtain the maximal

amount of information from the EST, a protocol can be altered somewhat to meet the clinical situation. The Bruce and the Ellestad protocols are shown below.

Table 3.2
Exercise Stress Test Protocols

Bruce Protocol:

| 3 min | 1.75 mph | 10% grade |
|-------|----------|-----------|
| 3 "   | 2.5  "   | 12%   "   |
| 3 "   | 3.4  "   | 14%   "   |
| 3 "   | 4.2  "   | 16%   "   |
| 3 "   | 5.0  "   | 18%   "   |

Ellestad Protocol:

| 3 min | 1.6 mph | 10% grade |
|-------|---------|-----------|
| 2 "   | 2.2  "  | 10%   "   |
| 2 "   | 2.6  "  | 10%   "   |
| 2 "   | 3.0  "  | 10%   "   |
| 2 "   | 3.6  "  | 10%   "   |

2.  **ECG Monitoring in EST.** If a single lead is to be used for ECG monitoring in EST, **lead V5** usually provides the largest R wave and, therefore, the greatest likelihood for detecting ECG changes. Sensitivity is enhanced by 15% by using a **12-lead ECG** system which also detects ST segment changes from the anterior and inferior walls(Figure 3.1)(4).

ECGs are routinely done supine and standing prior to the EST, at each step in the EST protocol, immediately postexercise, and at 2-min intervals thereafter for 10 min.

## INTERPRETATION

1.  ST segment changes are the most reliable electrocardiographic indicators of myocardial ischemia.  **Six major types of ST segments may occur in response to exercise** (Figure 3.2).

2.  A horizontal or down-sloping ST segment which is depressed at least 1 mm below the isoelectric at the J point and which persists for 80 msec thereafter is interpreted as a positive test (see figure 3.2 patterns C and D).  The **incidence of false positives is significantly reduced** when a 2-mm ST segment depression requirement

is used for a positive test. Three consecutive beats without baseline variation are required for reliable measurement of ST segments. Two examples of a positive EST are shown in Figures 3.1 and 3.3.

3. The **depth of the ST segment depression correlates roughly with the extent of coronary artery disease,** i.e., patients with 3-mm or greater ST segment depression 80 msec after the J point have a high incidence of triple vessel disease. In addition, ST segment changes which occur in the first 3 min of exercise and/or persist past 8 min during recovery correlate with an 85% prevalance of two and three vessel disease(5).

4. Other patterns of ST segment depression (see figure 3.2):

    **Pattern B.** Depression of the J point with a rapid rise in the ST segment is a normal occurrence with exercise and correlates poorly with IHD.

    **Pattern E.** Depression of the J point with a slow-rising ST segment and 2.0-mm ST depression at 80 msec from the J point has been shown to correlate well with IHD, but there is a high incidence of false positives (32%). Therefore, this pattern is not widely used for the diagnosis of IHD.

    **Pattern F.** ST segment elevation occurs rarely in EST and probably represents a severe degree of myocardial ischemia, or an LV aneurysm(6). No quantitative criteria are established for EST interpretation.

5. Interpretation of the EST must also include:

    - An evaluation of the workload performed.

    - The heart rate and BP response.

    - The presence or absence of arrhythmias.

    - The presence or absence of symptoms.

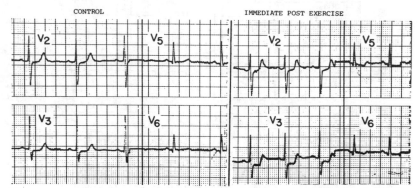

**Figure 3.1   Control and Immediate Postexercise ECGs in a Patient with IHD**

Note the 2-mm horizontal ST segment depression in lead V3. This diagnostic change would not have been detected if only lead V5 had been monitored.

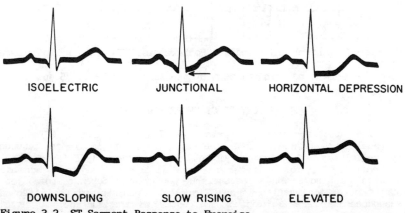

**Figure 3.2   ST Segment Response to Exercise**

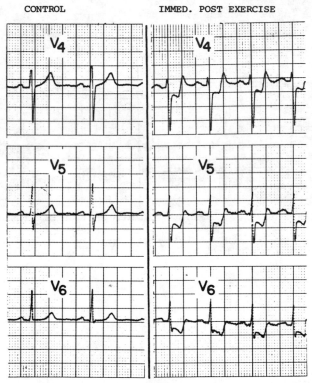

CONTROL                    IMMED. POST EXERCISE

**Figure 3.3  Control and Immediate Postexercise ECGs in a Patient with IHD**
Note the 3-mm downsloping ST segment depression in leads V5 and V6.

## PHYSIOLOGY OF ST SEGMENT DEPRESSION

The **electrophysiologic basis for ST changes during EST** is an intracellular potassium loss resulting from an imbalance between myocardial oxygen supply and demand.  The subendocardial layer of the left ventricle is most vulnerable because it is subjected to a high wall tension which adversely affects tissue perfusion.  Subendocardial loss of potassium ion results in an ST segment shift toward the affected subendocardial area, which is manifested on the surface ECG as ST depression.

## OTHER CAUSES OF ST SEGMENT DEPRESSION

1. **Supply/demand imbalance** due to anemia, aortic stenosis, coronary spasm, severe hypertension, left ventricular hypertrophy, hypertrophic cardiomyopathy.

2. **Left bundle branch block.** Induces secondary repolarization changes unrelated to supply/demand imbalance.

3. **Drugs.** Digitalis (this drug is usually discontinued 10 days prior to the EST if atrial fibrillation is not present), antihypertensives.

4. **Miscellaneous.** Cardiomyopathies, mitral valve prolapse, Syndrome X (chest pain with angiographically normal coronary arteries).

5. **Hypokalemia, recent glucose or food ingestion, vasoregulatory asthenia.**

## JUST HOW WELL DOES EST PREDICT IHD?

**The predictive value of any test will vary with the prevalence of the disease in the population being tested.** Thus, the greater number of patients with IHD in the population being tested, the greater the predictive value. Therefore, populations tested with few risk factors for IHD will have a larger number of false-positive responses and a decreased predictive value. Females of any age have a high incidence of false positive tests as compared to males of the same age group(7).

1. Summary of 15 studies using ST segment depression alone (1 mm, patterns C and D) as an indicator of IHD in populations referred for evaluation.

   **Sensitivity** = 64%    (Percent that EST correctly identified as patients having IHD from a group of patients known to have IHD)

   **Specificity** = 85%    (Those patients with negative tests who are truly normal)

   **Predictive**
   **Value**    = 80%    (Likelihood of IHD if EST is positive)

2. Results are also influenced by the severity of CAD present; for example, only 9% of patients with triple vessel disease had false-negative tests, whereas 63% of patients with single vessel disease had a false-negative EST.

## COMMON MISCONCEPTIONS ABOUT EST

1. EST is the definitive tool to verify the existence of IHD.

   POINT:  Overall sensitivity is 64%; therefore, 36% of patients with CAD will have a false negative test.

2. There is little benefit from the EST in subjects with known IHD, especially those considered stable post-MI.

   POINT:  The treadmill may be used to determine those patients at high risk for future coronary events: i.e., a patient with a positive EST 2 months post-MI is twice as likely to have a future coronary event as a patient with a negative EST post-MI(2,8).

   POINT:  EST is used to establish efficacy of drugs (antianginal agents/antiarrhythmics) and to establish an exercise prescription in cardiac rehabilitation programs.

3. ST segment depression is the only manifestation of IHD.

   POINT:  Many other aspects of EST may correlate with the presence and severity of IHD.  Look for:

   A. Submaximal pulse response (chronotropic incompetence correlates with LV dysfunction)(2).

   B. Fall in blood pressure(9).

   C. Exercise-induced chest pain(10).

   D. Ventricular ectopy(11).

   E. Magnitude and configuration of ST segment depression(5).

   F. Time of onset of ST segment depression, i.e., earlier onset correlates with more severe disease(5).

   G. Length of time ST segment abnormalities persist in recovery phase; longer-lasting abnormalities correlate with more severe disease(5).

# REFERENCES

1.  Rochimis P, Blackburn H: Exercise tests: A survey of procedures, safety, and litigation of experience in approximately 170,000 tests. JAMA 217:1061, 1971.

2.  Ellestad MH: Stress Testing: Principles and practice. Philadelphia, F.A. Davis Company, 1975.

3.  Bruce RA, Hornsten TR: Exercise testing in the evaluation of patients with ischemic heart disease. Prog Cardiovasc Dis 11:371, 1969.

4.  Chaitman BR, Bourassa GB, Wagniart P, et al: Improved efficiency of treadmill exercise testing using a multiple lead ECG system and basic hemodynamic exercise response. Circulation 57:71, 1978.

5.  Goldschlager N, Selzer A, Cohn K: Treadmill stress tests as indicators of presence and severity of coronary artery disease. Ann Intern Med 85:277, 1976.

6.  Chahine RA, Raizner AE, Ishimori T: The clinical significance of exercise induced ST-segment elevation. Circulation 54:209, 1976.

7.  Linhart JW: Maximum treadmill exercise electrocardiography in female patients. Circulation 50:1173, 1974.

8.  Markiewicz W, Houston N, DeBusk RF: Exercise testing soon after myocardial infarction. Circulation 56:26, 1977.

9.  Levites R, Baker T, Anderson GJ: The significance of hypotension developing during treadmill exercise testing. Am Heart J 95:747, 1978.

10. Weiner DA, McCabe C, Hueter DC, et al: The predictive value of anginal chest pain as an indicator of coronary disease during exercise testing. Am Heart J 96:458, 1978.

11. Udall JA, Ellestad MH: Predictive implications of ventricular premature contractions associated with treadmill stress testing. Circulation 56:985, 1977.

Chapter 4

# Echocardiography

The development of echocardiography in the past two decades has been a major advance in the noninvasive evaluation of cardiac conditions. A knowledge of the capabilities and limitations of echocardiography is a must for all clinicians who interpret, or even request, echocardiograms(1).

## PRINCIPLES OF ULTRASOUND

Ultrasound is sound energy at a frequency above the level of human perception. Medical imaging ultrasound, however, lies only in a narrow frequency range of ultrasound (2 to 10 MHz) that combines the best in resolution but still allows for adequate penetration of tissue. Higher-frequency ultrasound would yield better resolution but would penetrate tissue only a short distance and vice versa for low-frequency ultrasound. Ultrasound waves are both transmitted and received by a transducer on the chest wall. The generated ultrasound waves are reflected back to the transducer by the interface between two tissues of different acoustical impedance such as myocardium or a valve and blood. The strongest echoes and, therefore, the best images are achieved when the reflected surface is perpendicular to the ultrasound beam. **Ultrasound does not travel well through air, so it cannot penetrate lung tissue.** This accounts for the poor echocardiograms obtained in patients with obstructive lung disease since the lung can overlie a part or all of the heart. **Ultrasound also does not penetrate bone, which limits the usefulness of echocardiography in the presence of chest wall deformities.**

## EXAMINATION OF THE NORMAL HEART

A complete echocardiographic evaluation can include all four types of examination: M-mode, two-dimensional, Doppler, and contrast echocardiography. Each of these will be described in detail.

## M-MODE ECHOCARDIOGRAPHY

The M-mode or "one-dimensional" echocardiogram is actually two dimensions: distance from the transducer is recorded on the vertical axis and time is recorded on the horizontal axis. **The M-mode study requires 3 transducer positions** (Zones 1, 2, and 3 in Figure 4.1).

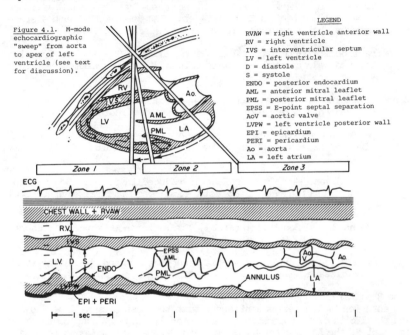

Figure 4.1. M-mode echocardiographic "sweep" from aorta to apex of left ventricle (see text for discussion).

LEGEND

RVAW = right ventricle anterior wall
RV = right ventricle
IVS = interventricular septum
LV = left ventricle
D = diastole
S = systole
ENDO = posterior endocardium
AML = anterior mitral leaflet
PML = posterior mitral leaflet
EPSS = E-point septal separation
AoV = aortic valve
LVPW = left ventricle posterior wall
EPI = epicardium
PERI = pericardium
Ao = aorta
LA = left atrium

**Zone 1** is used to obtain measurements of ventricular dimensions and thickness of the walls. From anterior (ventral) to posterior (dorsal), the measurements that are commonly obtained are:

**Right Ventricular Free Wall.** This measurement is often not seen well in adults.

**Right Ventricular Cavity (RV).** This measurement roughly correlates with RV volume.

**Interventricular Septum (IVS).** Septal movement is normally posterior during systole and anterior in diastole. A paradoxical septal motion implies a RV volume overload or a conduction abnormality such as left bundle branch block. Septal thickness can also be used to evaluate hypertrophy.

**Left Ventricular (LV) Cavity.** Measurements of the LV cavity are made at end-diastole (onset of QRS complex of ECG) and end-systole (at maximum anterior motion of the posterior wall). These measurements roughly correlate with LV volume in diastole and in systole.

**Pericardium.** Normally there is no echo-free space between the epicardial and pericardial surfaces. The presence of such a space suggests that a pericardial effusion is present.

**Fractional Shortening.** This is an index of ejection fraction obtained by LV diastolic diameter minus LV systolic diameter divided by LV diastolic diameter.

**Zone** 2 contains the mitral valve (MV) apparatus (Figure 4.2). Values obtained from this orientation of the transducer include:

**Opening Excursion.** This is an index of the mobility of the mitral valve and is also influenced by the rate and volume of diastolic inflow.

**E to F Slope.** This measurement is reduced in patients with a slow inflow across the MV during diastole, as seen in mitral stenosis or a hypertrophic, noncompliant left ventricle.

**E Point–Septal Separation (EPSS).** This distance, which is measured between the fully opened anterior mitral leaflet and the IVS correlates **inversely** with angiographic ejection fraction. The correlation is invalid in aortic regurgitation and rheumatic mitral valve disease.

**Zone** 3 contains the aorta (Ao), aortic valve (AoV), and left atrium (LA). The anterior MV leaflet is continuous with the posterior wall of the Ao, and the IVS is continuous with the anterior Ao. The RV outflow tract is in front of the Ao, and the LA is behind the Ao. Measurements in Zone 3 include:

**Aortic (Ao) Root.** The aorta is seen as a series of parallel lines that move anteriorly with systole.

**Aortic Valve (AoV).** M-mode echocardiograms show 2 of the 3 leaflets opening during systole to almost the size of the Ao, and then closing during diastole to form a single line.

**Left Atrium (LA).** It is measured from the back wall of the Ao to the posterior wall of the LA at end-systole. As a general rule, the LA is approximately the same size as the Ao.

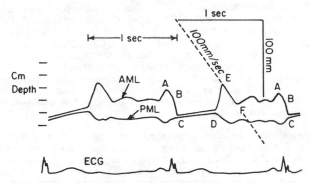

**Figure 4.2  Normal Echocardiographic Mitral Valve Motion**
The  upward excursion of the anterior mitral leaflet (AML) resulting from
atrial systole forms the **A point,** which correlates with the "a" wave in
the left atrial pressure.  The mitral closure point is C, which
correlates with left atrial "c" waves.  There may be a shoulder between A
and C, designated **B.**  The gradually up-sloping **C to D** line represents the
closed valve moving apically and anteriorly during ventricular systole
(descent of the base).  The **D to E** excursion is the mitral opening, and
the **E to F** excursion represents the valve "floating" towards closure after
the rapid ventricular filling period.  Depending on the length of
diastole, there is a variable distance and often several undesignated
undulations between **F** and the next **A** point.

The values for normal M-mode echocardiographic measurements are
given in Table 4.1(2).  Some echocardiography laboratories normalize
these values for body size.

**Table 4.1**
**Normal M-Mode Measurements**

| | |
|---|---|
| RV (diastole) | <2.5 cm |
| LV (diastole) | <5.5 cm |
| LV (systole) | Variable |
| Septum | <1.2 cm |
| Posterior Wall | <1.2 cm |
| EPSS | <0.5 cm |
| EF Slope | 50-150 mm |
| Fractional Shortening | 20-50% |
| Aortic Valve Opening | >1.7 cm |
| Aortic Root | <3.8 cm |
| Left Atrium | <4.0 cm |

## TWO-DIMENSIONAL ECHOCARDIOGRAPHY

The use of two-dimensional (2D) echocardiography gives important anatomical information not available on M-mode examination, Although M-mode echocardiograms are used to obtain standard measurements of structures, 2D echocardiography is better at estimating chamber volumes, especially if there are segmental wall motion abnormalities. Two-dimensional echocardiography can also measure MV area and is better than M-mode echocardiography at detecting vegetations. Two-dimensional echocardiograms are usually recorded on videotape. Most systems now are capable of recording both **M-mode and 2D images--the two methods are complimentary and not exclusive.**

The transducer positions necessary for a complete examination are dependent on the patient's anatomy and anatomic areas of interest. **Minimal views should include:** parasternal long axis, parasternal short axis (with multiple "slices" from apex to aorta), and apical four-chamber. Additional views that are usually recorded include subcostal, apical two-chamber (LA and LV), and suprasternal notch.

## DOPPLER ECHOCARDIOGRAPHY

Doppler echocardiography uses the principle that the frequency of a reflected sound wave depends on the velocity of the flowing blood and the angle of impact by the ultrasound waves on the blood elements. The difference between the emitted and the measured frequencies is termed the Doppler shift. In Doppler echocardiography, the reflected surface is usually the moving red blood cells, so that **velocity and direction of blood flow can be** estimated and in some cases precisely measured. Instead of continuously transmitting and recording Doppler signal (continuous wave), one can pulse the ultrasound (pulse wave) to allow simultaneous Doppler and 2D echocardiography. This has the advantage of allowing localization of a Doppler "sample" in the area of interest, but it cannot correctly measure high velocities. The Doppler signal is most often displayed as a spectrum of flow velocities to show either laminar or turbulent flow and direction of flow (toward the transducer it is above the baseline and away from the transducer it is below the baseline). Recent work has shown good correlation between Doppler - derived transvalvular gradient and cardiac catheterization data in patients with mitral or aortic stenosis. The presence and severity of valvular regurgitation can also be estimated by Doppler echocardiography. It is also used to detect intracardiac shunts in congenital heart disease.

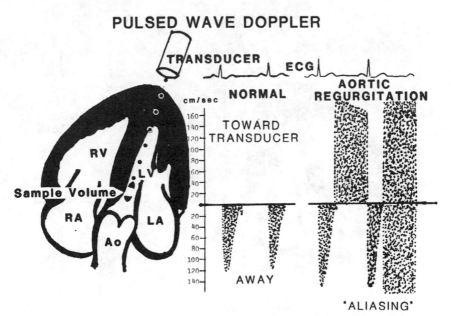

**Figure 4.3   Pulsed-Wave Doppler**
The transducer has been aimed along the long axis of the left ventricle
from the cardiac apex, and the "sample volume," or sampling depth, is
denoted by the space between the two semicircles within the outflow tract.
In the example of normal flow, only outflow away from the transducer is
seen at about 120 cm/sec or 1.2 m/sec.   In the example of aortic regurgitation, there is higher- velocity systolic outflow and a regurgitant
flow toward the transducer.   In the last cardiac cycle, the velocity of
regurgitant flow has exceeded the Nyquist limit of the pulsed-wave
Doppler system, and there is "aliasing" or a wraparound flow signal that
appears to be going toward and away from the transducer.   When the Nyquist
limit is exceeded, the true velocity and direction of flow cannot be
determined with pulsed-wave Doppler, and continuous-wave Doppler must be
used.

# CONTINUOUS WAVE DOPPLER

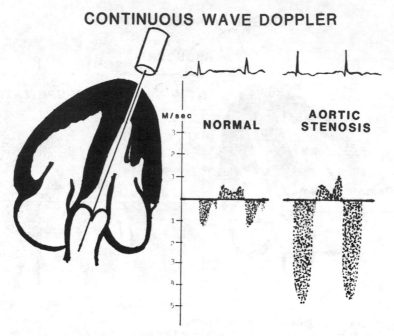

**Figure 4.4    Continuous-Wave Doppler**

The transducer has been aimed along the long axis of the ventricle and records all flow patterns that are encountered, since a sample volume cannot be set as in pulsed-wave Doppler (see Figure 4.3). In the normal example, flow velocities are seen representing aortic outflow (away from the transducer) during systole and mitral inflow (toward the transducer) during diastole. In aortic stenosis, the outflow velocity is higher than normal, and the flow pattern is more rounded, symmetrical, and longer lasting. The transvalvar gradient can be calculated from the Bernoulli equation, or 4 multiplied by the square of the velocity, as over 90 mm Hg.

## CONTRAST ECHOCARDIOGRAPHY

The injection of almost any liquid, such as blood, saline, or indocyanine green dye, into the intravascular space will produce tiny microbubbles that appear as a very bright echo-dense cloud on the echocardiogram. **This can be a sensitive method of determining right-to-left shunts** such as atrial or ventricular septal defects(4). An example is shown in Figure 4.12.

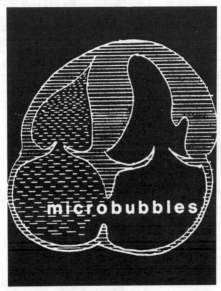

**Figure 4.5    Contrast Echocardiography**
Injections of indocyanine green dye, saline, or blood cause microbubbles which are echo-dense and act as contrast media.   The microbubbles do not traverse the pulmonary capillaries, so intravenous injections remain in the right heart chambers unless there is a right-to-left shunt.

---

Certain cardiac diseases have classical echocardiographic findings. Some of the more common disease states are presented in the following examples.

### ECHOCARDIOGRAPHY IN VALVULAR HEART DISEASE

#### Rheumatic Mitral Valve Disease

Mitral valve (MV) disease on echocardiography is characterized by:
1) thickened MV leaflets with commissural fusion, 2) decreased E-F slope,
and 3) anterior motion of both the anterior and posterior MV leaflets
during diastole (Figure 4.6A).  If stenosis is the predominant lesion,
the LA is large and LV size is normal to small.  If mitral regurgitation
is predominant, the LV and LA are large with exaggerated wall motion (LV
and LA volume overload state).  The LA is almost always enlarged.
**Doppler echocardiography is very sensitive for detecting MR.**  The degree
of regurgitation is assessed by determining how far into the LA the
regurgitant echoes are detected.  Doppler echocardiography can estimate
MV gradient by measuring MV inflow velocity (pressure gradient = $4V^2$,
where V = maximal velocity).

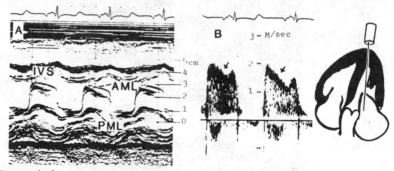

**Figure 4.6    Rheumatic Mitral Valve Disease**
(A) M-mode echocardiogram through the MV that shows a thickened mitral
valve, reduced E to F slope, and diastolic anterior motion of the
posterior mitral valve leaflet (PML).  IVS is the intraventricular
septum and AML is the anterior mitral leaflet.  (B) Continuous-wave
Doppler recording which depicts the high flow of 2 m/sec (arrow) through
the MV during diastole that represents flow toward the transducer (i.e.,
toward the apex).  The mitral valve gradient can be estimated by:

$$4V^2 = 16 \text{ mm Hg}.$$

#### Aortic Stenosis

Aortic stenosis (AS) is seen as thickening of AoV leaflets and
decreased AoV opening (Figure 4.7A).  Secondary effects on the LV include
hypertrophy, prolonged emptying of the LV, and, in the later stages of AS,
LV dilatation.  Doppler echocardiography can measure a pressure gradient
across the AoV to  determine the severity of disease(5) (Figure 4.7B).

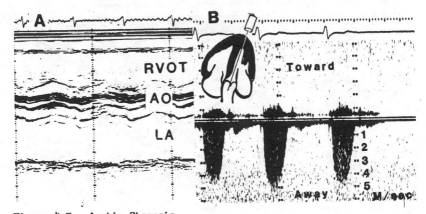

**Figure 4.7    Aortic Stenosis**
(A) M-mode view through the AoV that shows thickened leaflets that do not open perceptibly with systole.  The LA is enlarged (4.5 cm).
(B) Continuous-wave Doppler recording with an apical transducer position demonstrates high velocity flow (3 m/sec) away from the transducer.

## Aortic Regurgitation

Direct detection of aortic regurgitation (AR) is not made by conventional echocardiography.  However, the causes of AR may be detected, such as an endocarditis, dissection, or flail leaflet.  The most common and sensitive indirect M-mode sign of AR is fine diastolic fluttering of the anterior MV leaflet or septum due to the regurgitant flow from the Ao into the LV(6) (Figure 4.8A).  Preclosure of the MV before the onset of ventricular systole is a sign of severe, usually acute AR(7).  LV volume overload (LV dilation and exaggerated wall motion) is also consistent with moderate to severe AR.  Doppler echocardiography can detect AR when the sample volume in the LV outflow tract detects turbulent flow in diastole toward the apical transducer (Figure 4.8B).

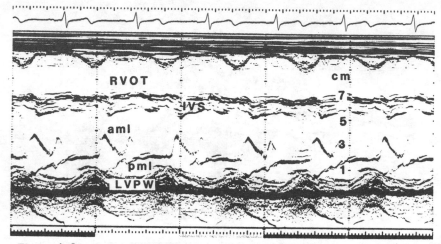

**Figure 4.8A  Aortic Regurgitation**
M-mode echocardiogram through the MV showing the fine diastolic
fluttering of the anterior mitral valve leaflet (AML).

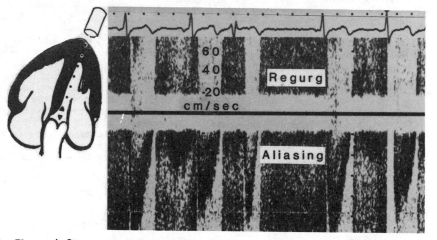

**Figure 4.8B  Aortic Regurgitation**
Pulsed-wave Doppler recording from an apical port shows regurgitant flow
toward the transducer during diastole and aortic outflow during systole.
The velocity of regurgitant flow exceeds the Nyquist limit and "aliasing"
is seen.

## Mitral Valve Prolapse

Mitral valve prolapse (MVP) is one of the most frequent reasons for referral for echocardiography. Unfortunately, **there is no consensus on the exact criteria for the diagnosis.** Late systolic dorsal excursion of the MV leaflet on the M-mode echocardiogram is the most specific sign of MVP (Figure 4.9). On 2D echocardiograms, one or both MV leaflets should traverse the plane of the mitral annulus during systole. Thickened or redundant MV leaflets are an echocardiographic sign of clinically important MVP. The complications of severe MVP can also be seen on the echocardiogram: endocarditis, flail leaflet, or mitral regurgitation by Doppler.

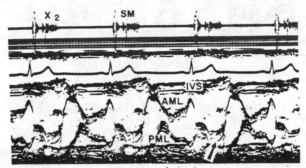

**Figure 4.9    Phonoechocardiogram of Mitral Valve Prolapse**
The free-swinging AML impacts on the IVS in early diastole and then meets the elongated PML in mid-diastole. Shortly after normal systolic apposition of the leaflets, a posterior bowing of both leaflets is seen (arrow). The nadir of this posterior movement coincides with 2 mid-systolic clicks (X) and the beginning of a late systolic murmur (SM).

## Infective Endocarditis

Infective endocarditis (IE) is more readily diagnosed by 2D than by M-mode echocardiography. Absence of vegetations, unfortunately, does not exclude the diagnosis of IE(8). Very large vegetations are often due to fungal disease (Figure 4.10). Since vegetations persist after bacteriological cure of endocarditis, the presence of vegetations does not necessarily indicate active endocarditis.

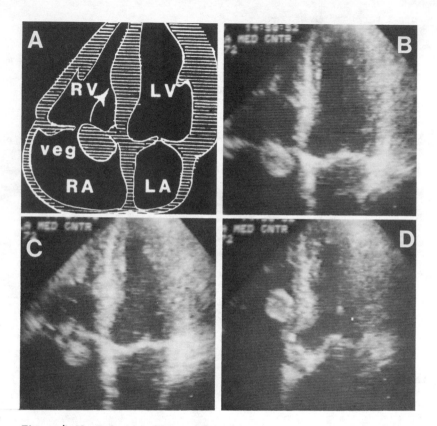

**Figure 4.10   Infective Endocarditis**
Two-dimensional echocardiography in the **apical 4-chamber** view
demonstrates a large mobile vegetation attached to the septal leaflet of
the tricuspid valve. (A) A diagram depicts the vegetation (veg) in
systole, and its diastolic motion is indicated by the arrow. (B) A
systolic frame corresponding to the diagram demonstrates the vegetation
in the right atrium. (C) An early diastolic frame shows the sling-like
attachment to the tip of the septal leaflet as the vegetation is being
flung toward the right ventricular cavity. (D) The vegetation is in the
right ventricle, adjacent to the interventricular septum in mid-
diastole.

## ECHOCARDIOGRAPHY IN CARDIOMYOPATHIES

### Dilated Cardiomyopathy

The echocardiogram in patients with dilated cardiomyopathy (DCM) shows a diffusely dilated, poorly contractile LV. M-mode signs of a reduced stroke volume include a reduced MV opening and gradual closure of the AoV. The normally smooth A-C slope in the M-mode echocardiogram of the MV can have a "B notch" which correlates with an elevated end-diastolic pressure (Figure 4.11). LV volume is usually increased. Left ventricular mural thrombi are frequently demonstrated.

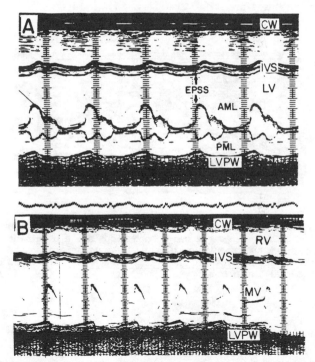

**Figure 4.11  Dilated Cardiomyopathy**
(A) The mitral valve is suspended in a large cavity; there is a large E-point septal separation (EPSS = 2.8 cm). (B) Both ventricles are enlarged and there is poor wall motion.

## Hypertrophic Cardiomyopathy

Hypertrophic cardiomyopathy (HCM) has characteristic findings on an echocardiogram: 1) usually asymmetric septal hypertrophy (septal to posterior wall thickness ratio of >1.5), 2) systolic anterior motion (SAM) of the anterior leaflet of the MV, 3) normal or increased ejection fraction, and 4) mid-systolic closure of the aortic valve leaflets(9) (Figure 4.12). The cavity of the ventricle is small in diastole and may obliterate in systole as a result of exaggerated excursions of the LV walls.

**Figure 4.12   Hypertrophic Cardiomyopathy**
Three echocardiographic views of a patient with typical HCM. The diagnostic features are underlined:

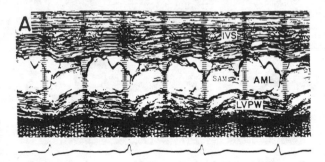

A.  **Zone** 2 demonstrates a mitral valve situated anterior to the usual location which impinges on the thickened IVS in diastole and systole. There is a reduced E to F slope and a prominent "a" wave because of the poorly compliant left ventricle. After mitral closure there is systolic anterior movement of both mitral leaflets with septal impingement.

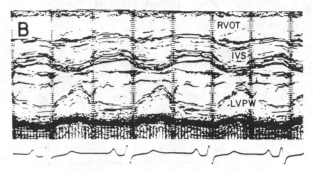

B. **Zone 1** demonstrates the asymmetrically thickened LV walls (LVPW = 1.4 cm, IVS = 2.6 cm, IVS/LVPW = 1.8) and the small LV cavity which is nearly obliterated during systole. The excursion of the LVPW is more pronounced than the IVS.

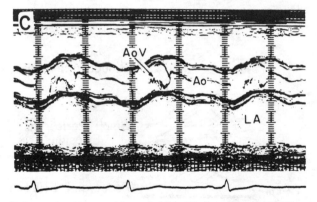

C. **Zone 3** demonstrates a mid-systolic closing motion of the posterior cusp of the aortic valve (AoV) denoted by the arrow. The left atrium is enlarged (5 cm).

### ECHOCARDIOGRAPHY IN MISCELLANEOUS CONDITIONS

**Pericardial Effusion**

Pericardial effusion (PE) is detected on the echocardiogram when there is an echo-free space between the epicardial and pericardial surfaces(10)  (Figures 4.13 and 4.14).  It is considered large if there is also an anterior echo free space.  The heart will "swing" within a large PE and give rise to electrical alternans (see Chapter 14, Pericardial Heart Disease).

## Pericardial Effusion

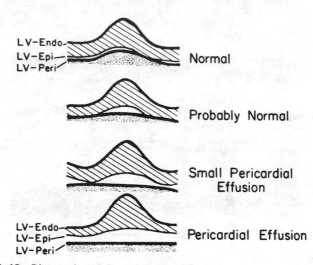

**Figure 4.13  Diagnosis of Pericardial Effusion**
A "clear space" between the epicardium and pericardium which is present during diastole **and** systole is necessary for accurate diagnosis of a pericardial effusion.

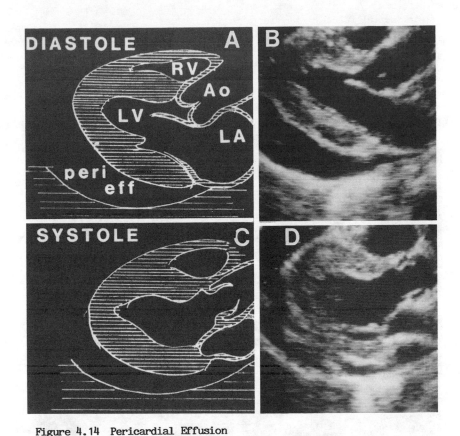

**Figure 4.14 Pericardial Effusion**
Two-dimensional echocardiography in the **parasternal long axis** view
(corresponding to Figure 4.1) in a patient with a large pericardial
effusion with tamponade demonstrates an echo-free space behind the left
ventricle which represents the pericardial effusion (peri eff). (A) A
diagram depicting the diastolic appearance of the heart with the anterior
leaflet approaching the interventricular septum and the aortic valve
closed. (B) This diastolic frame corresponds to (A). (C) A diagram
depicting the heart in systole, with the mitral valve closed and the
aortic valve open. Systolic collapse of the left atrium is seen as an
indentation of the posterior atrial wall. (D) This systolic frame
corresponds with (C). A rocking motion of the heart can be appreciated by
noting the ventral position of the heart in diastole and the dorsal
position in systole.

## Atrial Septal Defect

Atrial septal defect (ASD) can often be diagnosed by direct visualization of the defect, especially in the subcostal view.  However, echo "dropout" may give the false impression of an ASD.  More importantly, one should see the effects of an ASD:  RV enlargement and paradoxical septal motion.  Contrast echocardiography (Figure 4.5) will demonstrate a "negative contrast" effect as blood without bubbles moves from the LA to the bubble-filled RA via the ASD.  Since there is usually some degree of right-to-left shunt in most patients with an ASD, bubbles will be seen in the left-sided chambers as well (Figure 4.15).

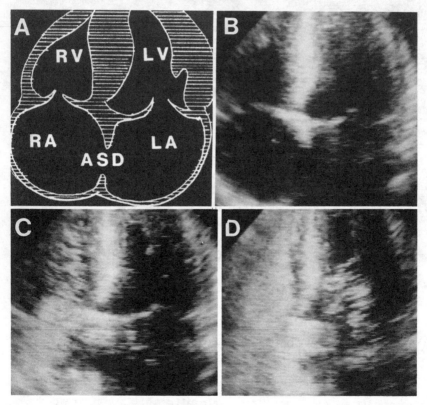

**Figure 4.15  Atrial Septal Defect**
Two-dimensional  echocardiography  in  the  **apical  4-chamber**  view demonstrates a large ASD.  (A) A diagram demonstrates the location of the cardiac  chambers  and  the  echo  dropout  in  the  mid-atrial  septum

suggesting an ASD. (B) This echo frame corresponds to (A). (C) Immediately after an antecubital vein injection of indocyanine green dye, a cloud of echo-dense microbubbles fills the right heart chambers, and a negative washout (encroachment of echo-lucent blood into the microbubbles) is seen in the region of the ASD, demonstrating a left-to-right shunt. (D) A later frame after the injection of microbubbles demonstrates right-to-left shunting into the left atrium and left ventricle.

## REFERENCES

1. Popp RL: Echocardiographic assessment of cardiac disease. Circulation 54:538, 1976.

2. Sahn DJ, DeMaria A, Kisslo J, et al.: The Committee on M-mode Standardization of the American Society of Echocardiography. Circulation 58:1072, 1978.

3. Henry WL, DeMaria A, Gramiak R, et al.: Report of the American Society of Echocardiography on nomenclature and standards in two-dimensional echocardiography. Circulation 62:212, 1978.

4. Seward JB, Tajik AJ, Hagler DJ, et al.: Peripheral venous contrast echocardiography. Am J Cardiol 39:202, 1977.

5. Hatle L, Angelsen BA, Tromsdal A: Noninvasive assessment of aortic stenosis by Doppler ultrasound. Br Heart J 43:284, 1980.

6. Skorton DJ, Child JS, Perloff JK: Accuracy of the echocardiographic diagnosis of aortic regurgitation. Am J Med 69:377, 1980.

7. Botvnick EH, Schiller NB, Wickramasekaran R, et al.: Echocardiographic demonstrations of early mitral valve closure in severe aortic insufficiency: Its clinical implications. Circulation 51:836, 1975.

8. Mintz GS, Kotler MN, Segal BL, et al.: Comparison of two-dimensional and M-mode echocardiography in the evaluation of patients with infective endocarditis. Am J Cardiol 43:738, 1979.

9. Rossen RM, Goodman DJ, Inghma RE, et al.: Echocardiographic criteria in the diagnosis of idiopathic hypertrophic subaortic stenosis. Circulation 50:747, 1974.

10. Horowitz MS, Schultz CS, Stinson EB, et al.: Sensitivity and specificity of echocardiographic diagnosis of pericardial effusion. Circulation 50:239, 1974.

# Chapter 5

# Nuclear Cardiology

In the last ten years, nuclear cardiology has developed rapid, accurate, noninvasive means for evaluating regional myocardial perfusion and quantitating cardiovascular performance. The technical advances that have made this possible include the availability of appropriate radiopharmaceutical agents, high-performance gamma-scintillation cameras, and low-cost computer equipment which allows rapid data acquisition and analysis. The noninvasive nature of these techniques has resulted in widespread applicability and acceptance(1).

All nuclear cardiology procedures can be separated into three broad categories:

1.  Myocardial perfusion imaging.

2.  Infarct avid imaging.

3.  Radionuclide angiography.

Myocardial perfusion imaging assesses myocardial blood **flow** by using radiopharmaceutical agents which are injected into the blood stream and accumulate in the myocardium. Thallium-201 is a radioisotope which is delivered to all organs of the body in relative proportion to the blood flow each organ receives. The heart accumulates thallium-201 in areas of viable myocardium in proportion to blood flow to those regions. The greater the perfusion of blood to a region of the myocardium, the greater the uptake of thallium-201 to that region. Regions with decreased blood flow are represented by decreased or absent thallium uptake and are seen as "cold spots."

The most widely used clinical applications for myocardial perfusion imaging is stress testing with thallium-201. During this procedure, the patient undergoes stress testing with an IV line in place. Approximately 1 min before stopping exercise, thallium-201 is injected intravenously and soon thereafter the patient is taken to the nuclear medicine department where the gamma-scintillation camera is used to image the myocardium (stress phase). In areas of decreased myocardial blood flow, diminished uptake of thallium-201 is noted(2). If repeat images are obtained 3 or 4 hours later at rest (redistribution phase), changes from the stress images will reflect changes in regional myocardial blood flow occurring with exercise. Thus, cold spots which are seen with maximal exercise and disappear with rest, indicate regions of the myocardium that have decreased blood flow with exercise but adequate blood flow at rest. Areas of reversible hypoperfusion, corresponding to reversible ischemia, indicate areas of significant obstructions to coronary artery blood flow. The standard treadmill stress test has about a 50-60% specificity depending on the population under study. A thallium-201 stress test has a specificity of over 90%. A negative thallium-201 stress test makes the diagnosis of significant coronary artery disease very unlikely. The sensitivity of the thallium-201 stress testing is over 85%. In contrast, the sensitivity of standard ECG treadmill testing is about 50-70%.

Thallium "cold spot" imaging is useful in a number of conditions, including:

1.  Diagnosis of coronary artery disease, particularly in patients with a conflicting data base (e.g., suspected false-positive stress ECG, false-negative stress ECG with a convincing history for angina, patients with pre-existing ECG abnormalities such as left bundle branch block [LBBB], digitalis therapy, left ventricular hypertrophy [LVH], etc.).

2.  Evaluation of patency of coronary artery bypass grafts, particularly in patients with chest pain after bypass surgery(3).

3.  Determination of the physiologic significance of coronary artery stenosis discovered by coronary angiography.

4.  Detection of additionally jeopardized myocardium after a myocardial infarction suggesting multivessel coronary artery disease.

5.  Acute myocardial infarction can be diagnosed, sized, and localized with an accuracy approaching 100% if a resting thallium study is done within 6 hours of the onset of symptoms(4). Cold spot defect resolution strongly suggests coronary artery spasm. Small infarcts, subendocardial infarcts, and scans performed later than 24 hours after the onset of symptoms can all result in negative scans.

6.  Patients with **right ventricular pressure overload** (pulmonic valve stenosis or pulmonary hypertension) as well as patients with **right ventricular volume overload** (left-to-right intra-cardiac shunts or tricuspid stenosis) will have a diagnostic thallium-201 scan. In normal resting thallium-201 scans, the right ventricle usually is not visualized due to its thin wall

and low regional blood flow.  With right ventricle pressure or volume overload the right ventricle works harder, resulting in right ventricular hypertrophy and increased regional blood flow to the right ventricle.  Increased blood flow results in increased thallium-201 uptake, and the right ventricle is visualized in the resting image(5).

7.   Patients with dilated cardiomyopathy may have characteristic thallium-201 scans.  Patients with ischemic disease as an etiology for their dilated cardiomyopathy typically demonstrate multiple large perfusion defects.  In contrast, patients with idiopathic dilated cardiomyopathy generally have homogeneous uptake of thallium-201 in the myocardium.

8.   Patients with sarcoidosis and myocardial involvement will have thallium-201 scans with multiple patchy left ventricular perfusion defects.

The second type of myocardial imaging is the infarct avid imaging or **technetium pyrophosphate scan**.  Pyrophosphate forms complexes with deposits of calcium.  Infarction results in the influx of calcium and phosphate ions.  In infarcted areas interaction of the pyrophosphate and calcium occurs in the damaged myocardial tissue and is subsequently detected as a "hot spot" when viewed with a gamma camera(6).  The central area of an infarct typically has very reduced blood flow and, therefore, deposition of the radiopharmaceutical pyrophosphate is less than that in the peripheral areas.  This results in a so-called "doughnut" pattern of pyrophosphate deposition, with a central area with almost no pyrophosphate uptake as a result of very low flow at the center of the infarct and a circular surrounding zone of high uptake corresponding to the peripheral areas of the infarct with lesser reductions in coronary blood flow(7).

Pyrophosphate is normally used as a bone imaging agent, and a normal pyrophosphate scan image demonstrates no activity in the region of the heart, with activity seen best in the ribs, sternum, and vertebral column. A positive pyrophosphate scan results in one of two types of uptake:

1.   Focal uptake in one anatomic region of the heart.

2.   Diffuse uptake in the entire heart not limited to any specific anatomic region.

Patients can be imaged at the bedside using a portable camera. Maximal uptake of pyrophosphate occurs between 48 and 72 hours and most scans revert to normal in 7 to 17 days(6).

Occasionally, scans can remain persistently positive for weeks or months, possibly related to ongoing cellular necrosis or aneurysm formation(8).

Transmural infarcts result in a positive scan in over 90% of cases if imaging is performed 2 to 3 days after infarction. Nontransmural, subendocardial infarctions are detected less frequently (perhaps 50% of the time)(9).

Acute myocardial infarction is the most common cause for a positive technetium pyrophosphate scan, but there are a number of other conditions which infrequently can result in a positive scan, including:

1. Left ventricular aneurysms.

2. Myocardial contusions.

3. Valvular calcifications (thought to be due to pyrophosphate binding to calcium).

4. Cardiomyopathy (diffuse uptake).

5. Unstable angina pectoris (diffuse uptake).

Technetium pyrophosphate scanning is often useful in conditions which suggest myocardial infarction but where the usual noninvasive tools are not helpful. Examples include:

1. After cardiac or other forms of surgery where high levels of creatine kinase will be present. The pyrophosphate scan can determine whether or not infarction has occurred.

2. Atypical chest pain in patients with equivocal ECG or enzyme changes.

3. Patients with chest pain and ECGs which do not allow assessment of transmural injury (e.g., LBBB).

4. Patients with pre-existing infarcts and evidence for infarct extension.

5. Myocardial contusion.

The third class of nuclear cardiology procedures is radionuclide angiography, sometimes called radionuclide ventriculography. This technique allows visualization of the atria and ventricles utilizing radioactive **intravascular** indicators to create pictures of the great vessels and chambers of the heart.

There are two types of radionuclide ventriculography:  The first-pass method and the gated equilibrium method.  In the first-pass method a bolus of a technetium compound, e.g., technetium sodium pertechnetate, is injected intravenously and sequential cardiac images are obtained at a rapid rate   during the initial passage of the radiotracer through the great vessels and chambers of the heart.   The tracer first passes through the superior vena cava and the right-sided chambers of the heart.   Since the tracer moves through the lungs rapidly, good separation of the right and left heart chambers can be achieved.   Background activity is minimized because most of the radiopharmaceutical is in the heart itself during imaging.   The first-pass study can be done rapidly(10).

Utilizing the gated equilibrium method of blood pool imaging, red blood cells are labeled with technetium, which allows imaging of the heart chambers and can be repeated many times.   Gating means obtaining a repetitive image of the heart at a predetermined time after the onset of the QRS complex.   Each cardiac cycle is divided into a series of segments by the computer, and tracer counts from corresponding segments of the cardiac cycle from multiple heart beats are added together to create one summed picture of the cardiac chambers at one set time in the cardiac cycle.   This allows for an averaged picture of the cardiac chambers from diastole to systole.

The gated method allows the calculation of end-systolic and end-diastolic counts.   Therefore, calculation of left and right ventricular ejection fractions can be performed using the formal end-diastolic counts minus end-systolic counts (stroke count) divided by end-diastolic counts.   The ejection fractions so calculated are highly correlated with values obtained by standard contrast ventriculography at cardiac catheterizations.

Regional wall motion abnormalities can be detected by displaying the end-diastolic  and end-systolic images in a static format.   In addition, sequential frames of the cardiac cycle can be displayed on a video monitor to create a "movie" of ventricular function over an entire cardiac cycle.   This helps in the precise localization of regional wall motion abnormalities.

Ventricular volumes can be determined using data from gated radionuclide ventriculograms.   Geometric formulas usually used with routine contrast ventriculograms have been utilized to approximate ventricular volumes.   A more common technique for volume determination compares the isotope **activity** in a known volume of the patient's blood drawn at the time of the radionuclide ventriculogram.   This allows conversion of isotope counts in the ventricle to volume in the ventricle.

**A priori,** the right ventricular (RV) stroke volume and left ventricular stroke volume should be equal.   In the presence of aortic regurgitation (AR) or mitral regurgitation (MR), however, left ventricular stroke volume will be greater than right ventricular stroke volume and the difference will represent the **regurgitation fraction.**

Left ventricular aneurysms can be detected utilizing radionuclide ventriculography. Left ventricular aneurysms result in a paradoxical image with end-systolic images protruding beyond end-diastolic images and the regional difference representing aneurysmal dilatation.

Right ventricular ejection fractions can be calculated from both first-pass and gated studies. Radionuclide ventriculograms revealing dilatation of the right ventricle and a reduced RV ejection fraction are seen in right ventricular infarcts.

In normal hearts, exercise results in an increase in the left ventricular ejection fraction. On the other hand, coronary artery disease results in a decline or no change in ejection fraction with exercise. Radionuclide ventriculography detects this decrease in ejection fraction, as well as regional wall motion abnormalities with exercise. The sensitivity of exercise radionuclide ventriculography for detecting coronary disease is better than utilizing exercise electrocardiography alone and is similar to exercise thallium-201 scans(11). The specificity of the technique is similar to that of the stress ECG. Advantages of radionuclide ventriculography include a lower cost for technetium 99m than for thallium-201 and the ability of radionuclide ventriculography to assess ventricular function, information thallium scans cannot provide. Disadvantages include the requirement for computer acquisition and processing of the study information.

Radionuclide ventriculography provides useful information about chronic valvular heart disease, particularly regarding aortic and mitral regurgitation. These data may be useful in the timing of valve replacement surgery. Compensated regurgitant lesions (AR, MR) result in an increased stroke volume. There is an increased end-diastolic volume with a normal end-systolic volume. With time, chronic valvular regurgitant lesions result in progressive dysfunction of the left ventricle marked by a decrease in resting ejection fraction and failure to increase ejection fraction with exercise. In addition, an increase in end-systolic volume is seen. These very sensitive indicators of worsening left ventricular function may be of value in assessing a patient's need for valve replacement(12).

The first-pass method of radionuclide ventriculography can accurately predict the presence and extent of left-to-right cardiac shunts. A technetium compound is injected into the external jugular vein and followed as it passes through the right heart, the lungs, and then through the left heart. A computer-derived region of interest is placed over the lung and the computer plots the counts that occur in that region over time. In normal patients, the pulmonary time-activity curve shows an initial peak as the tracer moves through the lungs, followed by a later smaller secondary peak due to "recirculation" as part of the tracer bolus reappears in the lungs after having traveled through the systemic circulation. A left-to-right intracardiac shunt results in the early and prominent reappearance of the secondary peak curve because of the early reappearance of the tracer that took a "short cut" through the shunt back to the right heart rather than the longer route through the systemic circulation. A normal shunt study effectively excludes an intracardiac left- to-right shunt of any clinical significance.

Right-to-left shunts may be detected by early appearance of tracer in the left-sided chambers or in the aorta.

## REFERENCES

1. Berger HJ, Zaret BL:  Nuclear cardiology (Part 1).  N Engl J Med 305:799, 1981.  Nuclear cardiology (Part 2).  N Engl J Med 305:855, 1981.

2. Richie JL, Trobraugh GB, Hamilton GW, et al.:  Myocardial imaging with thallium-201 at rest and during exercise.  Circulation 56:66, 1977.

3. Ritchie JL, Narahara KA, Trobaugh GB, et al.:  Thallium-201 myocardial imaging before and after coronary revascularization: Assessment of regional myocardial blood flow and graft patency. Circulation 56:830, 1977.

4. Wackers FJ Th, Sokole EB, Samson G, et al.:  Value and limitations of thallium-201 scintigraphy in the acute phase of myocardial infarction.  N Engl J Med 295:1, 1976.

5. Cohen HA, Baird MG, Rouleau JR, et al.:  Thallium 201 myocardial imaging in patients with pulmonary hypertension.  Circulation 54:790, 1976.

6. Parkey RW, Bonte FJ, Meyer SL, et al.:  A new method for radionuclide imaging of acute myocardial infarction in humans.  Circulation 50:540, 1974.

7. Rude RE, Parkey RW, Bonte FJ, et al.:  Clinical implications of the technetium-99m stannous pyrophosphate myocardial scintigraphic "doughnut" pattern in patients with acute myocardial infarcts. Circulation 59:721, 1979.

8. Malin FR, Rollo D, Gertz EW:  Sequential myocardial scintigraphy with technetium-99m stannous pyrophosphate following myocardial infarction.  J Nucl Med 19:1111, 1978

9. Prasquier R, Taradesh MR, Botvinick EH, et al.:  Specificity of the diffuse pattern of cardiac uptake in myocardial infarction imaging with technetium 99m stannous pyrophosphate.  Circulation 55:61, 1977.

10.  Reduto LA, Berger HJ, Cohen LS, et al.:   Sequential radionuclide
     assessment of left and right ventricular performance after acute
     transmural myocardial infarction.   Ann Intern Med 89:441, 1978.

11.  Jengo JA, Oren V, Conant R, et al.:   Effects of maximal exercise
     stress on left ventricular function in patients with coronary artery
     disease using first pass radionuclide angiocardiography.   A rapid,
     noninvasive  technique  for  determining  ejection  fraction  and
     segmental wall motion.   Circulation 59:60, 1979.

12.  Borer  JS,  Bacharach  SL,  Green  MV,  et  al.:   Exercise  induced
     ventricular dysfunction in symptomatic and asymptomatic patients
     with  aortic  regurgitation:   Assessment  with  radionuclide  cine-
     angiography.   Am J Cardiol 42:351, 1979.

# Chapter 6

# Cardiac Catheterization

Many cardiac problems can be properly diagnosed and treated without the need for invasive procedures. In some clinical situations, cardiac catheterization may be required to manage the cardiac patient. **The decision to study a patient invasively is one that should be carefully considered.** The clinician must take into consideration the clinical setting, the patient's age, and past medical and/or surgical history of the suspected cardiac problem. The individual performing the procedure is, in fact, performing a high-level consultation and not merely a laboratory test. He or she should have a thorough knowledge of the patient and, most importantly, what questions must be answered by the procedure in the specific patient undergoing study.

Before the patient consents to an invasive study, he or she must be informed of the **risks of the procedure.** Although the risks vary depending on the type of case, cardiac catheterization in a stable patient is very safe with competent personnel and carries with it a less than 1% probability of morbidity. The risks are amplified in more elderly or more infirm patients and in patients who are not physiologically or psychologically stable at the time of the procedure. An extensive review of complications of coronary angiography showed the risk of myocardial infarction to be 0.13%, stroke to be 0.006%, and overall death rate to be 0.19% in over 14,000 cases(1). Other complications include local thrombosis, embolism, bleeding, cardiac perforation, significant arrhythmias, and allergy to contrast media.

The referring physician should be satisfied that the procedure can be done safely and adequately and that the laboratory has the ability to answer the clinical questions. Not all catheterization laboratories are properly equipped with a wide range of laboratory equipment and not all catheterization personnel have adequate training and experience.

**Patients with ischemic heart disease** constitute the majority of cases in the average cardiac catheterization laboratory. The principal information needed in these cases is an angiographic demonstration of the nature and extent of disease in the coronary arteries, the left ventricular filling pressure, ejection fraction, size, wall motion, and valvular competence.  **Patients with congenital or valvular heart disease** require more elaborate physiologic studies in order to identify the anatomical relationships, pressures, and regional blood flow in the central circulation(2,3).

The **two methods of vascular access** are the Seldinger percutaneous technique (utilizing the femoral vein and/or artery) and surgical exposure or cut-down of the brachial vessels.  There is no appreciable difference in complications between the two approaches for experienced laboratories.  Advantages of the transfemoral approach include the greater likelihood of traversing an atrial septal defect or patent foramen ovale and the ability to use the transseptal technique if the left atrium must be entered or if prosthetic heart valves preclude retrograde access to the left heart.

A procedure which has been used with increasing frequency in recent years is **percutaneous transluminal coronary angioplasty (PTCA),** in which arterial stenoses are dilated by balloon inflation.  Initially, this procedure was limited to single-vessel lesions in coronary artery disease (CAD) patients who were symptomatic on medical treatment.  Presently, a much broader spectrum of patients is undergoing this nonsurgical technique, including those with multivessel CAD, patients with previous coronary artery bypass grafting (CABG) surgery and stenosis in the native or graft vessels, patients with acute myocardial infarction (MI) who present very early in their course to a properly equipped facility, and certain high-risk surgical cases (elderly patients with renal failure, systemic diseases, and some with severe left ventricular dysfunction).

In experienced hands, PTCA is a low-risk procedure with 1% or less mortality and approximately 5 to 10% morbidity(4) including MI, arrhythmia, infection, bleeding, and the need for emergency CABG because of dissection or acute closure (5).  The success rate for experienced operators is 80 to 90% per vessel dilated.  Certain advantages of PTCA make it an attractive alternative to surgery; e.g., it is less expensive and does not necessitate general anesthesia and thoracotomy, and duration of hospitalization is shorter.  At this time the major pitfall of PTCA is restenosis, which occurs in approximately 20% of cases within the first year.  These recurrent stenoses can be redilated 90% of the time.  The long-term fate of lesions dilated by PTCA is an important but yet unanswered question.

**Electrophysiologic studies** are performed in relatively few properly equipped laboratories.  These invasive procedures involve placing multipolar catheter electrodes into various cardiac chambers for the purpose of stimulating or recording potentials from the atria, ventricles, and the His bundle.  Candidates for this procedure include those with refractory or life-threatening supraventricular or ventricular tachycardias, survivors of sudden cardiac death, patients with unexplained syncope, and patients with atrioventricular accessory pathways(6).  With pacing of the atria or ventricle and introduction of premature extrastimuli, supraventricular and ventricular tachycardias can be induced in the majority of patients who have these clinically significant arrhythmias.  Induction of a tachycardia is useful both in elucidating its mechanism and in choosing a treatment strategy.  A drug that suppresses a previously inducible tachyarrhythmia has a high possibility of preventing spontaneous episodes of the arrhythmia. Similarly, a drug that does not prevent inducibility is unlikely to be clinically effective.

In situations where drug therapy is ineffective, it is possible, using several multipolar pacing electrodes, to "map" the site of origin of a tachyarrhythmia or to precisely localize the position of an atrioventricular bypass tract.  These areas can then sometimes be ablated, either surgically or via catheter-delivered electrocautery.

A thorough review of the terminology and physiologic data derived from cardiac catheterization is beyond the scope of this text.  However, a table of normal values is included for the reader's reference.

## Table 6.1
## Normal Values and Pressures

### Normal Values

| | |
|---|---|
| $O_2$ consumption ($VO_2$) | $110-150/ml/min/M^2$ |
| Pulmonary arteriovenous (AV)$O_2$ difference | 3.5–4.7 vol.% |
| Systemic AV $O_2$ difference | 3.5–4.7 vol.% |
| Systemic $O_2$ saturation | $\geq 94\%$ |
| Cardiac index (CI) | $2.5-4.0$ L/min/$M^2$ |
| Systemic vascular resistance (SVR) | 8.0–15.0 units |
| Pulmonary vascular resistance (PVR) | 0.2–1.12 units |
| Total pulmonary resistance (TPR) | 1.0–3.0 units |
| Aortic valve area (AVA) | $2.6-3.5$ cm$^2$ |
| Mitral valve area (MVA) | $4.0-6.0$ cm$^2$ |
| Left ventricular (LV) end-diastolic volume | <90 ml/$M^2$ |
| Ejection fraction | 55–70% |
| His bundle electrogram AH interval | 60–115 msec |
| HV interval | 35–55 msec |

**Normal pressures** (mm Hg)

| | |
|---|---|
| Right atrium (RA), mean | 1-8 |
| Right ventricle (RV) systolic | 15-28 |
| End-diastolic (RVEDP) | 0-8 |
| Pulmonary artery (PA) | |
|   Systolic | 15-28 |
|   Diastolic | 5-16 |
|   Mean | 10-22 |
| Pulmonary artery wedge (PAW) | |
|   Mean | 4-12 |
| Left atrium (LA) | |
|   Mean | 4-12 |
| Left ventricle (LV) | |
|   Systolic | 85-150 |
|   End-diastolic (LVEDP) | 4-12 |
| Aortic (Ao) | |
|   Systolic | 85-150 |
|   Diastolic | 60-90 |
|   Mean | 70-105 |

## REFERENCES

1. Hansing CE: The risk and cost of coronary angiography. JAMA 242:735, 1979.

2. Criley JM, French WJ: Cardiac catheterization in adults with congenital heart disease. In: Congenital Heart Disease in Adults. Cardiovascular Clinics, October 1979, p. 173.

3. Yang SS, Bentivoglio LG, Maranhao V, et al.: From Cardiac Catheterization Data to Hemodynamic Parameters. Philadelphia, F. A. Davis Company, 1978.

4. Gruntzig AR, Senning A, Siegenthaler W:  Nonoperative dilatation of coronary artery stenosis:  Percutaneous transluminal coronary angioplasty.  N Engl J Med 301:61, 1979.

5. Hartzler GO:  Coronary angioplasty:  Indications and results.  In Schroeder JS (ed):  Invasive Cardiology.  Cardiovascular Clinics. Philadelphia, F.A. Davis Co., 1985, pp.97-107..

6. Horowitz LN, Spielman SR, Greenspan AM, et al.:  Role of programmed stimulation in assessing vulnerability to ventricular arrhythmias. Am Heart J 103:604, 1982.

# Chapter 7

# Ischemic Heart Disease: General Considerations

The major clinical presentations of patients with coronary artery disease (CAD) are **angina, myocardial infarction, congestive heart failure,** or **sudden death.** Each of these is discussed in the chapters which follow.

## GENERAL COMMENTS

General facts about coronary artery disease have been derived from epidemiologic, laboratory, and clinicopathologic data(1):

1.  Coronary atherosclerosis is a multifactorial disease.

2.  The incidence and mortality of CAD increase with age, but atherosclerosis is not a necessary component of the aging process.

3.  The disease and its complications are more common in men than women. It is a rare disease in young white females, but it accounts for 35% of all deaths in men aged 55 to 64.

4.  There are marked cultural and ethnic variations in the incidence and mortality rate of CAD. Ischemic heart mortality for a 50-year-old American male living in the United States is five times greater than that of a 50-year-old native Japanese male living in Japan.

## RISK FACTORS

Seven major risk factors have been identified in association with CAD. It is of note that the risk of a coronary event in any individual rises exponentially when two or more major risk factors are present.

1.  **Age.** The incidence and mortality of CAD increases with age in both sexes.

2.  **Sex.** Males have a significantly higher risk of CAD than premenopausal females. After menopause, the incidence of CAD in females

approaches that of age-matched males.  Among Caucasian Americans, the male mortality rate from CAD is five times greater than females at ages 35-44.

3. **Family History.**  Patients with first degree relatives manifesting CAD before age 55 have a greater risk of developing coronary atherosclerosis.  Risk may be as high as five times the normal risk.

The next three risk factors are either modifiable or preventable:

4. **Cigarette Smoking**(2):  The risk of death from CAD is two to six times higher in smokers than in nonsmokers.  It has been estimated that the combination of birth control pills and smoking increases the incidence of coronary obstructive disease 30-fold.

5. **Hypertension.**  An estimated 60 million Americans have hypertension. Both systolic and diastolic pressure are risk factors, even in the elderly.

6. **Hyperlipidemia**(3,4).  Hypercholesterolemia has been conclusively shown to be a significant risk factor; the higher the level, the greater the risk.  On the other hand, studies of serum triglyceride levels have not conclusively shown correlation between increased levels and CAD.  The major plasma lipids, including cholesterol and triglycerides, are not in solution in the blood but are transported in the form of lipoprotein complexes--chylomicrons, very low-density lipoproteins (VLDL), low-density lipoproteins (LDL), and high-density lipoproteins (HDL).  LDL account for 60-75% of total cholesterol, and their blood level is directly related to the risk of CAD.  HDL account  for 20-25% of total cholesterol, and there is an inverse relationship between the level of HDL and atherosclerosis. Increased ("protective") levels of HDL are found in subjects who exercise, are not overweight, regularly eat a low carbohydrate diet, or have a modest intake of alcohol.

Five patterns of hyperlipoproteinemia have been described but only one (Type II) has been associated with increased risk of CAD.

| | |
|---|---|
| TYPE I | Increased chylomicrons |
| TYPE IIA | Increased LDL |
| TYPE IIB | Increased LDL and VLDL |
| TYPE III | Increased LDL |
| TYPE IV | Increased VLDL (principally triglycerides) |
| TYPE V | Increased chylomicrons and VLDL |

It is important to make a distinction between primary and secondary hyperlipidemias. Treatment of secondary hyperlipidemias is aimed at treating the underlying cause (such as diet, diabetes, myxedema, liver disease, renal disease, medications, alcoholism, porphyria, multiple myeloma).

Primary Type II (familial hypercholesterolemia) is inherited most commonly as an autosomal dominant trait and is associated with a high risk of developing premature vascular disease. Evidence suggests that this is a heterogeneous disorder. Clinical features include tendon xanthomas, premature corneal arcus, and xanthelasma. In the severe homozygous cases, CAD develops in childhood and patients rarely survive to adulthood without radical intervention.

Familial hypercholesterolemia is thought to result from a defect in cellular receptor mechanisms, with a failure to "turn off" the endogenous production of cholesterol, so that dietary restriction is relatively ineffective. Bile-acid binding resins, nicotinic acid, ileal bypass, and monthly plasma exchanges are the main therapeutic options.

7. **Diabetes**(5). Diabetics have two times the incidence of CAD as non-diabetics. Evidence suggests that strict control of blood sugar in patients with diabetes mellitus may retard or decrease the complications of CAD.

Other factors, such as sedentary lifestyle, personality type, obesity, and psychological tension may be contributing factors.

## RISK FACTOR MODIFICATION

Many physicians have tended to discount the significance of risk factors because attempts to modify them have not resulted in measurably increased survival. These disappointing results are due to the fact that medical interventions are often too little and too late(6). Coronary artery disease has a long latent period prior to the onset of symptoms of ischemia, so that the disease is often far advanced before it is recognized by the patient or the physician. Our philosophy is, therefore, to try to modify the risk factors to the best of our ability, recognizing that the patient may, in turn, positively influence others at an earlier stage of disease, particularly his or her children.

## NATURAL HISTORY

A comprehensive and meaningful study of the natural history of CAD has not been done; therefore, our knowledge is, by necessity, based on biased data. It is known that extensive CAD can be asymptomatic, and it is thought that there is often a long latency period, probably years and possibly decades, before obstructive lesions may become clinically manifest.   Because knowledge of coronary artery anatomy requires either postmortem examination or coronary arteriography, our data base, therefore, is skewed toward those with fatal or morbid complications.   On the other hand, not all CAD is insidious.   Dynamic changes in coronary luminal patency due to vasomotion, platelet plugs, thrombi, or subintimal hemorrhage can precipitate instantaneous symptoms and/or death.

The relevance of those facts that we do have is further confounded by the perturbations imposed by rapidly evolving therapeutic interventions, both pharmaceutical and mechanical.

Of the studies available, it is evident that the natural history of CAD is **primarily dependent** on the **status of the left ventricle** and, to a lesser degree, on the extent of coronary involvement(7).   The earlier survival data for patients with one, two, and three vessel disease projecting an increasingly grim prognosis has given way to steadily improving medical survival data from large prospective cooperative studies.   The marked improvement in prognosis is partially attributable to the more intelligent use of hygienic measures, patient education, and medical therapy, but other factors such as pre-hospital emergency cardiac care systems and the overall decline in heart disease death rate all contribute.

## REFERENCES

1.   Stamler J:   Epidemiology of coronary heart disease.   Med Clin North Am 59:5, 1973.

2.   Auerbah O, Hammond EC, Garfinkel L:   Smoking in relation to atherosclerosis of the coronary arteries.   N Engl J Med 273:775, 1965.

3.   Castelli WP, Doyle JT, Gordon T, et al.:   HDL cholesterol and other lipids in coronary heart disease.   Circulation 55:756, 1977.

4.   Kannel WB, Castelli WP, Gordon T, et al.:   Serum cholesterol, lipoproteins, and the risk of coronary heart disease:   The Framingham Study.   Ann Intern Med 74:1, 1971.

5.   Bradley RF, Partamian JO:   Coronary heart disease in the diabetic patient.   Med Clin North Am 49:1093, 1965.

6.   Borhani NO:   Primary prevention of coronary heart disease:   A critique.   Am J Cardiol 40:251, 1977.

7.   Nelson GR, Cohn PF, Gorlin R:   Prognosis in medically treated coronary artery disease:   Influence of the ejection fraction compared with other parameters.   Circulation 52:408, 1975.

# Chapter 8

# Angina Pectoris

Angina pectoris results from an imbalance between myocardial oxygen supply and demand and is most commonly caused by the inability of atherosclerotic coronary arteries to perfuse the heart under conditions of increased myocardial oxygen consumption (demand). Angina also occurs in patients with seemingly normal coronary arteries[1] subjected to acute or chronic increases in myocardial work such as aortic stenosis, hypertension, or hypertrophic cardiomyopathy. Coronary artery spasm, superimposed upon normal or diseased arteries, can provoke pain in the absence of increased myocardial demands and has been shown to be responsible for variant (Prinzmetal's) angina and certain cases of unstable angina. Lastly, there is a sizeable group of patients who have angina without evidence of coronary artery disease, with or without an increase in myocardial work. This latter syndrome has been termed "Syndrome X" because of its enigmatic nature.

## TYPICAL ANGINA PECTORIS (STABLE ANGINA)

**DESCRIPTION:**

**Character.** Most often described as a discomfort, pressure, heaviness, or squeezing sensation, and not a pain. Less commonly described as burning or sharp.

**Location.** Most often in the substernal area, precordium, or epigastrium with radiation to the left arm, jaw, or neck. Less commonly felt only in radiation areas and not in the chest.

**Precipitation.** Often provoked by exertion, emotion, cold weather, eating, or smoking, and relieved by rest, removal of provoking factors, or sublingual nitrates.

**Duration.** Usually lasts a few minutes, rarely over 30 minutes.

## EVALUATION:

**History.** The diagnosis of angina pectoris (AP) is established by obtaining a reliable description of the chest discomfort and its relationship to activity. The likelihood of underlying coronary artery disease is enhanced by a history of hypertension, diabetes mellitus, hyperlipidemia, smoking, or a family history of **premature** ischemic heart disease in first-degree relatives (age $\leq$ 55 years).

**Physical Examination.** Although often normal, examination may yield important confirmatory information, i.e., hypertension, peripheral arterial disease, xanthelasma, tendenous xanthomata, tobacco-stained fingers or teeth, or diagonally creased earlobes. Episodic ischemia alters left ventricular compliance and may produce papillary muscle dysfunction. A transient S4 and/or apical systolic murmur during angina or exertion are not uncommon.

**Blood Chemistry.** Basic screening is important to identify potentially treatable risk factors such as hypercholesterolemia and/or hyperglycemia. Hypertriglyceridemia is less well established as a risk factor. Elevated HDL (high-density lipoproteins) are a negative risk factor.

**Electrocardiogram.** Often normal in the absence of a myocardial infarction or a cause for left ventricular hypertrophy. An ECG during angina may show transient ST depression, T wave inversion, or ventricular arrhythmias.

**Exercise Stress Testing.** (EST; see Chapter 3). EST is invaluable in reproducing symptoms, documenting ischemic ECG changes, and assessing the level of disability. Patients with high-grade coronary artery disease may manifest inability to increase heart rate or blood pressure during exercise, or develop marked ST changes at low stress levels which persist after exercise. Exercise-induced arrhythmias or left ventricular dysfunction provide diagnostic information with important therapeutic potential. **Radionuclide scintigraphy** enhances the sensitivity and specificity of EST. Patients with significant coronary arterial obstructions will usually develop exercise-induced "cold spots" on thallium perfusion scanning or left ventricular wall motion abnormalities during nuclear scanning.

**Coronary Arteriography.** Although not necessary for diagnosis of coronary artery disease in most instances, cardiac catheterization and coronary angiography permit localization and quantification of obstructive lesions, evaluation of left ventricular function, and assessment of any valvular or myocardial disease. The **indications** for these invasive studies vary widely in different centers. Widely accepted indications include:

1.  Angina refractory to medical management.

2.  Angina or myocardial infarction in patients under 45 years of age.

3.  Unstable angina (after medical stabilization).

4.  Patients with persistent angina and/or low-level EST abnormalities after myocardial infarction.

5.  Marked (0.2 mV) ST changes at low-level exercise or persisting several minutes after cessation of EST.

6.  Suspected Prinzmetal's (variant) angina (coronary vasospasm).

7.  Preoperative evaluation of patients with valvular or congenital heart disease.

8.  Patients with life-threatening arrhythmias associated with ischemic heart disease.

9.  When needed for clarification of possible causes for recurrent chest pain when noninvasive testing has yielded negative or equivocal findings.

## GENERAL THERAPEUTIC CONSIDERATIONS:

**Risk Factor Reduction.**  Cessation of smoking, control of hypertension and diabetes, lowering cholesterol and lipids (usually by diet), and maintaining an ideal body weight are strongly advised.  The benefit of risk factor interventions **after** acute infarction has not been conclusively established.

**Exercise.**  The role of exercise in the treatment of patients with known ischemic heart disease remains controversial.  It has been established that regular exercise can lower the heart rate and blood pressure at rest and, during submaximal work loads, favorably modify the blood lipid composition, consume calories, and provide psychological benefits.  In certain patients, regular exercise may decrease cigarette smoking and result in more prudent eating habits.  However, the widely held concepts that exercise causes regression of coronary atherosclerosis, increases collateral formation, improves ventricular performance, and prolongs life lack rigorous scientific proof.  On the debit side, exercise causes an increase in the heart rate x blood pressure product, which increases myocardial oxygen demand.  Exercise can threaten the supply/demand balance of the myocardium and can produce ischemic dysfunction and arrhythmias in certain patients with latent or overt coronary artery disease.  Thus, a "prescription" for exercise must be written carefully with the knowledge of each individual patient taken into consideration.

**General Comments on Medical Therapy.** When medical therapy is indicated, the pharmacologic approach depends on the severity of the symptoms, side effect of the drugs, and the patient's response. Nitrates are very effective for acute relief, and long-acting nitrates should be the initial agent for maintenance therapy.

Medical therapy for angina patients has improved over the last decade. Optimal treatment with nitrates, beta blockers, and calcium blockers (a "stepped-care" approach) will result in marked improvement or complete relief of symptoms in many patients(2). Randomized clinical studies have shown improved long-term survival in patients with myocardial infarction treated with beta-blocking agents (propranolol, metoprolol, timolol)(3), as well as improved prognosis for patients with vasospastic angina treated with calcium-blocking agents. The trend in improved survival of patients with triple vessel disease (11.4% annual mortality in 1960s[4], 4.8% in VA study of the mid-1970s[5], and 2.1% in the recent CASS study[6]) is, in part, due to advances in pharmacologic therapy. Of interest, calcium blockers were not released prior to the initiation of the CASS study; it may be that their use will further improve long-term survival in patients with atherosclerotic ischemic heart disease.

## DRUG THERAPY—NITRATES:

**The mechanism of action** of nitrates in relieving angina is in large part due to a decrease in left ventricular work (by reducing venous return and preload, a determinant of myocardial oxygen demand) and to a lesser extent by coronary vasodilation and improved collateral flow.

**Short-Acting Sublingual Nitrates.** Sublingual nitroglycerin (0.4-0.3 mg or 1/150-1/200 gm) or isosorbide dinitrate (5-10 mg) is the most effective therapy for relieving an acute anginal attack, and may also be used prophylactically in anticipation of any angina-provoking activity. Relief is usually provided within 1 to 2 min, and the dose may be repeated within 5 min if the discomfort persists. The duration of action is about 2 hours.

**Oral Long-Acting Nitrates.** Since nitrates are degraded by the liver ("first-pass" metabolism), these long-acting oral preparations must be given in larger doses than the sublingual preparations. Isosorbide (10 to 40 mg P.O., q.i.d.) is an average effective dose range. **Therapy should be individualized** due to the variability of hepatic degradation.

**Topical 2% Nitroglycerin Ointment.** Absorbed slowly through the skin, it is especially effective in relieving nocturnal angina. An average dose is 1 to 2 inches (applied without rubbing into the skin) every 4 to 6 hours and covered with a nonabsorbing dressing. A terry cloth wristband, of the type worn by tennis players, provides an excellent retainer to cover the swatch of waxed paper used to dispense the drug. The therapeutic effectiveness of **nitroglycerin patches** in a fixed dose has been questioned. At present, this dosing technique offers no clear benefit or advantage and is not recommended.

**Contraindications.** Contraindications are hypersensitivity, hypotension, and hypovolemia. A relative contraindication may be severe nitrate-induced headaches, although the severity of headaches usually decreases with continued use of the drug.

## DRUG THERAPY—BETA-ADRENERGIC BLOCKING AGENTS:

These agents competitively occupy beta receptor myocardial sites (beta-1 receptors) and thus block the chronotropic and inotropic actions of catecholamines on the heart. In combination with nitrates, they can often prevent angina in a large percentage of patients with chronic stable angina. Noncardiac beta receptors (beta-2 receptors) in arterial walls and bronchial smooth muscle are also blocked by nonselective beta blockers.

### Nonselective Beta Blockers:

1. **Propranolol** (Inderal®) has had the longest record of clinical use of any of the currently available beta blocking agents in the United States and for this reason is widely used. The starting dose of Inderal is 10 to 20 mg P.O. t.i.d. or q.i.d. with stepwise increments as necessary to maintain the patient essentially angina free with normal daily activity. Total daily doses of 480 to 640 mg may be necessary in some cases. Although the resting heart rate may decrease to 50 beats per minute (bpm) with initial dosages, there is rarely a further fall with incremental doses. When a diuretic is required for management of hypertension in a patient with angina, Inderal may attenuate diuretic-induced potassium loss.

   Twice daily dosing of Inderal has been shown to be effective in relieving angina in many cases, as long as the same total 24-hour dose is maintained. Another alternative method is to use sustained-release Inderal with dosing on a once-a-day basis.

2. **Nadolol** (Corgard®) is a **long-acting** nonselective beta blocker which may be administered once a day, starting at 40 mg P.O. and progressing to 240 mg P.O. as needed.

3. **Timolol** (Blocadren®) is another newer nonselective drug which is usually started at 5-10 mg P.O. b.i.d. and increased up to 20 mg P.O. b.i.d.

## Cardioselective Beta Blockers.

1.  **Metoprolol** (Lopressor®) is a relatively cardioselective beta blocker at lower-dose ranges (less than 100 mg/day), and can be administered starting at 50 mg P.O. b.i.d., progressing as needed to 200-300 mg/day.

2.  **Atenolol** (Tenormin®) is a newer cardioselective blocker which is given once a day with starting dose of 50 mg and increased to 100 mg/day.

**Precautions and Contraindications.**  Overt **congestive heart failure** at rest is an absolute contraindication to the use of beta blockers because of the dependence of the failing myocardium on intrinsic adrenergic mechanisms.  **Severe bronchospasm** is an absolute contraindication to the use of nonselective beta blockers and a relative contraindiction to the use of selective beta-1 blockers.  **Insulin-dependent diabetes mellitus** is a relative contraindication to all beta blockers since the adrenergic response to hypoglycemia will be masked or blunted.

Many patients with chronic obstructive pulmonary disease (COPD), nonreversible airway obstruction due to emphysema, or well-controlled diabetes mellitus in combination with ischemic heart disease can tolerate and benefit greatly from beta blockers administered cautiously with close followup observation.  Similarly, patients with left ventricular dysfunction (ejection fraction 30 to 50%) which worsens with exercise can also benefit from cautious use of beta blockers since the myocardial supply/demand imbalance during exercise may be substantially decreased.

Noncardioselective beta blockers, by inhibiting beta-mediated arteriolar dilation, may worsen chest pain in some patients with coronary vasospasm and may be poorly tolerated by patients with severe peripheral arterial disease.  Systemic side effects in these patients at risk appear to be less with cardioselective blockers.

## DRUG THERAPY—CALCIUM-BLOCKING AGENTS:

Agents that inhibit channel calcium currents in cardiac and smooth muscle have been shown to be effective for relief or prevention of angina(7).

1.  **Nifedipine** (Procardia®) has been shown to be effective in increasing exercise tolerance and angina relief.  The starting dose is 10 mg P.O. t.i.d. or q.i.d., increasing as tolerated up to 30 mg P.O. q.i.d.  Symptoms related to hypotension can occur with any of the calcium blockers, although they are more frequent with Procardia.

Headache, dizziness, flushing, nausea, constipation, and dependent edema are common to all calcium blockers.

2. **Diltiazem** (Cardizem®) is started at 30-60 mg P.O. t.i.d. and increased up to 60-90 mg P.O. q.i.d.

3. **Verapamil** (Calan®, Isoptin®) is started at 80 mg P.O. b.i.d. and increased up to 120 mg P.O. q.i.d.

**Properties peculiar to each specific calcium blocker may be helpful in making a choice depending on clinical circumstances.** The hemodynamic effects of verapamil and diltiazem are similar to those of nonselective beta blockers (decreases in heart rate, decrease in arterial pressure, decrease in contractility). Effects of nifedipine are similar to those of nitrates (reflex increase in heart rate and reflex increase in contractility). Nifedipine appears to be a more potent arteriolar dilator than verapamil or diltiazem and thus is probably a preferable choice in patients with hypertension or CHF. Verapamil appears to have the most negative inotropic effects and is not well tolerated in patients with moderate to severe left ventricular dysfunction. Patients with recurrent symptomatic re-entrant supraventricular tachyarrhythmias would be better treated with verapamil or diltiazem. For those with sick sinus syndrome, nifedipine would be the best choice.

## PERCUTANEOUS TRANSLUMINAL CORONARY ANGIOPLASTY (PTCA)

PTCA is an effective treatment method for many patients with disabling symptoms and those with significantly jeopardized myocardium(8). PTCA has been used mainly in the treatment of single and select cases of double vessel disease and has recently been expanded to more complex cases with multivessel disease. PTCA is an attractive alternative to bypass surgery for many patients because of the decreased hospital time, major reduction in expense and minimal recovery time, and less operative insult. Relief of symptoms is usually seen in conjunction with objective improvement in exercise performance and improvement in ST changes. Restenosis continues to be a problem in approximately 20% of patients and is often heralded by recurrence of symptoms. Usually these patients can be redilated with a 90% success rate. An intimal tear in the balloon-dilated artery is also frequently encountered. This outcome is currently of uncertain importance in long-term effect.

## CORONARY ARTERY BYPASS GRAFTING (CABG):

Coronary revascularization can provide significant relief from angina to more than 80% of patients with angina refractory to drug therapy and has a low operative mortality (1-2%). It has, therefore, become a very common major operative procedure performed in the United States.

Since it neither reverses the disease process nor assures permanent revascularization, the use of the procedure should be limited to those patients who cannot be managed medically (risk factor modification, nitrates, beta blockers, and calcium channel blockers), those who have failed angioplasty, those found to have significant obstruction of the main left coronary artery, or significant obstruction (>70%) in all major arteries. Graft closure and recurrence of symptoms continues to be a problem with this form of therapy. The first year graft closure rate is 10-15%, and subsequently is 1-2% per year.

## UNSTABLE ANGINA PECTORIS

Unstable angina pectoris (UAP) is probably not a single entity, but a combination of syndromes which have been referred to by various names:

1. Preinfarction angina.

2. Crescendo angina.

3. Coronary insufficiency.

4. Angina decubitus.

DESCRIPTION:

The **character, location,** and **radiation** of chest discomfort in UAP may be similar to that of stable AP although it is often **more intense. UAP is distinguished from AP by the presence of one or more of the following criteria:**

**Precipitation.** May occur at rest or at a lower activity level compared to AP and may be less responsive to nitrates.

**Duration.** May last longer than AP, up to several hours in some cases.

**Frequency.** May occur more frequently than stable AP.

**ECG Changes.** More common than AP, UAP is often accompanied by reversible ECG changes of ischemia or injury. Such ECG changes may herald a poor long-term outcome (death due to a fatal cardiac event).

EVALUATION:

The evaluation of a patient with UAP should follow along the same lines as described in stable angina with the exception that **exercise stress testing (EST) should not be performed** until the patient has been clinically stable and free of pain for over 24 hours.   The presence of ECG changes of ischemia or injury during spontaneous UAP often precludes the necessity for EST.

## PATHOPHYSIOLOGY:

Like chronic stable AP, UAP often represents an imbalance between supply and demand; however, in UAP the level of demand is not always measurably increased.   Several mechanisms have been proposed to explain the pathophysiology(9):

1. Acute coronary thrombosis.

2. Platelet aggregation.

3. Coronary artery spasm.

4. Progression of atherosclerosis.

A report from the Montreal Heart Institute using serial angiographic studies over time (both before and after developing unstable symptoms) demonstrated **progressive coronary occlusion** in 75% of patients with unstable angina as opposed to 30% of a similar group of matched patients with stable angina(10). Although progression of athero- sclerosis may be a factor in developing unstable symptoms, a substantial percentage of patients have UAP symptoms without evidence of disease progression.

**Platelet aggregation** has been shown to be an important factor in experimental studies in the setting of partially occluded coronary arteries.   Pretreatment of dogs with aspirin before acute coronary occlusion has been shown to reduce the incidence of ventricular fibrillation and to increase  collateral blood flow(9).

Several studies have shown acute occlusion due to **intracoronary thrombosis** in a high percentage of UAP patients with fixed coronary obstruction(9).   In this regard, the effect of heparin on the development of transmural myocardial infarction (MI) in randomized patients with unstable angina has been studied.   Heparin significantly decreased the occurrence of acute MI, suggesting an important role of acute coronary thrombosis(11).

**Coronary spasm** superimposed on a fixed stenotic lesion may lead to total occlusion, infarction, and cardiac death(12).   It is unclear whether spasm alone can cause sufficiently severe ischemia to cause MI or if coronary vasospasm  results in localized platelet aggregation with intimal injury and thrombus formation.

## THERAPEUTIC CONSIDERATIONS:

Hospitalization with imposition of bed rest and sedation in an ECG-monitored environment is absolutely indicated in patients with UAP. Hypertension (if present) should be aggressively treated.

**Nitrates.** Sublingual nitroglycerin (0.4 mg) or isosorbide dinitrate (5 mg) should be administered for spontaneous episodes of pain with **monitoring of ECG and blood pressure changes** with pain and after nitrates. For long-acting nitrate therapy, topical nitroglycerin (2% ointment), 1 to 2 inches every 4 hours, is preferred to oral nitrates because of its more sustained effects. IV nitroglycerin may offer the most consistent relief of acute ischemia episodes and is often used in the more difficult cases. Starting dose is 0.5 mcg/kg/min and then increased as tolerated to control pain.

**Beta Blockers.** Beta blockers are administered in sufficient oral doses to achieve a resting heart rate between 50-60 bpm.

**Calcium Blockers.** Calcium blockers are routinely added to the medical therapy of unstable angina. These agents can be used as initial therapy along with nitrates or added to nitrates and beta blockers.

**Aspirin.** Since platelet aggregation has been strongly implicated in the pathogenesis of unstable angina and myocardial infarction, aspirin (a platelet inhibitor) was studied in a large Veterans Administration cooperative double-blind study to test whether endpoints of death and myocardial infarction were altered. The data showed a 51% lower incidence of myocardial infarction and death in the aspirin group (324 mg/day) as compared to the placebo group(13).

Aspirin causes irreversible acetylation of platelet cyclo-oxygenase, thereby preventing the formation of thromboxane $A_2$, an extremely potent vasoconstrictor and platelet activator.

Because of the above, it is presently our recommendation to add low-dose aspirin (75-mg baby size or 324-mg adult size) to the pharmacologic therapy of unstable angina.

## CLINICAL COURSE:

**Stable.** Most patients with UAP will respond to the medical therapy outlined above and can then be evaluated for extent of disability with the diagnostic tests outlined under stable angina pectoris. Our interpretation of prospective randomized series of medical versus medical plus surgical management of patients stabilized after UAP indicates that there is no urgency to proceed with coronary arteriography for consideration of immediate bypass surgery. There is no significant difference in mortality or myocardial infarction rate between the two groups.

However, more than 30% of the medically treated group eventually seek other methods of treatment(14).

**Unstable.** A small percentage of patients with UAP will fail to respond to medical management and will proceed to evolve a myocardial infarction. Another small percentage will remain unstable with unremitting pain. This latter group has a high incidence of eventual myocardial infarction with a high mortality(15), and it is our opinion that aggressive management is indicated as outlined below:

1.  Placement of flotation catheter for monitoring of wedge pressure and cardiac output.

2.  Use of intravenous nitroglycerin (0.5 to 2 mcg/kg/min) to control pain.   The goal should be to lower the wedge pressure to 15-20 mm Hg without inducing arterial hypotension or an increase in heart rate.

3.  If aggressive medical therapy is ineffective, intra-aortic balloon counter pulsation (IABP) should be tried.

4.  Coronary arteriography for consideration of emergent angioplasty or coronary bypass surgery can be done during IABP support.

## VARIANT ANGINA PECTORIS
### (PRINZMETAL'S ANGINA)

**DESCRIPTION:**

**Variant angina pectoris** (VAP) has also been termed **Prinzmetal's angina** and **angina inversa** because of its propensity to occur **at rest** and to be associated with **ST segment elevation,** which is the ECG inverse of typical AP. After the comprehensive clinical descriptions by Prinzmetal et al.(16) in the late 1950s and early 1960s, the first major breakthrough occurred in 1973 when Oliva demonstrated unequivocal **coronary artery spasm** associated with the pain and ST segment elevation of VAP(17). Subsequently, spasm has been seen in "normal" coronary arteries and those with fixed obstructions(12). Coronary artery spasm and VAP are probably not synonymous. Reversible spasm has been seen during unstable angina pectoris and early in the course of typical myocardial infarctions; it can be provoked by ergonovine stimulation in patients with obstructive coronary artery disease and typical AP(18).

**VAP is not a benign syndrome.** Myocardial infarction can occur in the region affected by coronary artery spasm in about 25% of patients and either high-grade heart block or ventricular fibrillation can occur during an episode of spasm. Although collective knowledge of the degree of overlap between the coronary spasm in VAP and that seen in "typical" CAD (AP or UAP) is incomplete, advancing a **diagnosis of VAP should be limited to those patients who fulfill two or more of the following criteria:**

1.  **Pain occurs principally at rest,** i.e., usually unprovoked(19). Since CAD may coexist, pain may also be provoked by exercise.

2.  **Pain may occur in a circadian manner,** i.e., recurrent episodes at a similar time of day, often in the early morning hours.

3.  **Pain is associated with ST segment elevation.** Often, subclinical (painless) episodes occur with "silent" ST segment elevations. Less commonly, **only ST segment depression** will occur (on a 12-lead ECG) in a patient who otherwise has typical VAP.

4.  **Painful or "silent" episodes are often associated with arrhythmias** --usually heart block and/or ventricular tachyarrhythmias or bundle branch block (including fascicular blocks).

## EVALUATION:

**History.**   The history of chest pain is often so atypical of ischemic heart disease as to be misconstrued by the physician as psychologic in nature, particularly since VAP is frequently seen in patients who have a paucity of risk factors.

**Electrocardiography.**   A 12-lead ECG during a spontaneous attack, demonstrating marked ST segment elevation, can establish the diagnosis with certainty.   In those patients with ST depression only, the diagnosis is less certain.   Since the episodes are often short lived and unpredictable, an ambulatory ECG (Holter) is statistically more likely to record the ECG changes; however, the limitation of conventional lead configurations may obscure the diagnostic features.

**Coronary Arteriography.**   Indicated in severely symptomatic patients with established or suspected VAP.   The goals of coronary arteriography should be to:

1.  Establish the status of the coronary vessels in an asymptomatic state.

2.  Establish the extent of change in the coronary arteries during spontaneous or induced (ergonovine) spasm.   A multilead ECG should be utilized to record simultaneous electrocardiographic and rhythm changes.

3.  Establish the response of spasm to sublingual nitrates.

## IMPORTANT CAVEATS IN VAP:

1.  Because patients with VAP may develop life-threatening arrhythmias, electromechanical dissociation, or profound spasm of major vessels

unresponsive to sublingual nitrates after ergonovine provocation, it is **not** advisable to utilize ergonovine stimulation outside a closely monitored setting.

2.  It is important to visualize both major coronary arteries during spontaneous or induced spasm since the surface ECG may reflect spasm of the more dominant artery (e.g., the right coronary artery) while another major artery branch (e.g., the left anterior descending coronary artery) is also in spasm.

## THERAPY:

**Nitrates.** Sublingual nitrates (nitroglycerin 0.4 mg or isosorbide dinitrate 5 mg) usually reverse spasm within 30-60 sec; oral nitrates (isosorbide dinitrate 20-40 mg every 4 hours) or topical nitrates can reduce the frequency of attacks. Since nitrates are **not** always successful and abrupt withdrawal of nitrates can provoke spasm in patients with seemingly normal coronary arteries, **it is important to taper and not to stop nitrates abruptly** regardless of their seeming ineffectiveness.

**Calcium Blockers.** Calcium blockers are extremely effective in preventing spasm in patients with VAP; use of these agents will generally result in marked reduction in frequency of episodes and need for nitroglycerin.

**Beta blockers are generally ineffective in VAP and have some theoretic disadvantages by blocking adrenergic coronary vasodilation.**

**Angioplasty or coronary bypass surgery is not effective in those patients with VAP without fixed lesions.** Selected cases with fixed underlying stenosis may need revascularization along with medical therapy.

## SYNDROME X

As noted in the introduction, there is a group of patients who have chest pain of seemingly ischemic origin but in whom neither CAD, VAP, or other evident cause for pain can be established. About 10% of patients with UAP and approximately 20% of patients thought to have typical AP have normal coronary arteriograms. These patients, for want of a better term, have been labeled as having **Syndrome X.** It is not known if the basis for the pain is a local metabolic imbalance, small vessel disease undetected by conventional coronary angiography, or a vasoregulatory disorder.

It is common practice to assume that there is a supply/demand imbalance in these patients and to treat them as though they had CAD. Prognosis is generally favorable.

## REFERENCES

1. Levine HJ: Mimics of coronary heart disease. Postgrad Med 64:58, 1978.

2. Chatterjee K, Rouleau JL, Parmley WW: Medical management of patients with angina. JAMA 252:1170, 1984.

3. Proceedings on the workshop on implication of recent beta-blocker trials for post-myocardial infarction patients. Circulation 67:I-1, 1983.

4. Reeves TJ, Oberman A, Jones WB, et al.: Natural history of angina pectoris. Am J Cardiol 33:423, 1974.

5. Murphy ML, Hultgren HN, Detre K, et al.: Treatment of chronic stable angina: A preliminary report of survival data of the randomized Veterans Administration Cooperative Study. N Engl J Med 297:621, 1977.

6. Coronary Artery Surgery Study (CASS): A randomized trial of coronary artery bypass surgery survival data. Circulation 68:939-50, 1983.

7. Pepine CJ, Feldman RL, Hill JA, et al.: Clinical outcome after treatment of rest angina with calcium blockers: Comparative experience during the initial year of therapy with diltiazem, nifedipine and verapamil. Am Heart J 106:1341, 1983.

8. Faxon DP, Detre KM, McCabe CH, et al.: Role of percutaneous transluminal coronary angioplasty in the treatment of unstable angina. Am J Cardiol 53:131C, 1984.

9. Epstein SE, Palmeri ST. Mechanisms contributing to precipitation of unstable angina and acute myocardial infarction: Implications regarding therapy. Am J Cardiol:54:1245, 1984.

10. Moise A, Theroux P, Taeymans Y, et al.: Unstable angina and progression of coronary atherosclerosis. N Engl J Med 309:685, 1983.

11. Telford AM, Wilson C: Trial of heparin vs. atenolol in prevention of myocardial infarction in intermediate coronary syndrome. Lancet 1:1224, 1981.

12. Hillis TD, Braunwald E: Coronary artery spasm. N Engl J Med 299:695, 1978.

13.  Lewis HD Jr, Davis JW, Archibald DG, et al.:  Protective effects of aspirin against acute myocardial infarction and death in men with unstable angina.  Results of a Veterans Administration Cooperative Study.  N Engl J Med 309:396, 1983.

14.  Becker LA, Giddle TL, Conti CR, et al.:  Unstable angina pectoris: National Cooperative Study Group to compare surgical and medical follow-up results in patients with one, two and three-vessel disease.  Am J Cardiol 42:839, 1978.

15.  Gazes PC, Mobley EM Jr, Faris HM Jr, et al.:  Preinfarctional (unstable) angina--prospective study--ten year follow-up. Prognostic significance of electrocardiographic changes.  Circulation 48:331, 1973.

16.  Prinzmetal M, Kennamer R, Merliss R, et al.:  Angina pectoris.  I. A variant form of angina pectoris.  Am J Med 27:375, 1959.

17.  Oliva PB, Potts DE, Pluss RG:  Coronary arterial spasm in Prinzmetal angina:  Documentation by coronary arteriography.  N Engl J Med 288:745, 1973.

18.  Heuler FA, Proudfit WL, Razavi M, et al.:  Ergonovine maleate provocative test for coronary arterial spasm.  Am J Cardiol 41:631, 1978.

19.  MacAlpin RN, Kattus AA, Alvard AB:  Angina pectoris at rest with preservation of exercise capacity:  Prinzmetal's variant angina. Circulation 47:946, 1973.

# Chapter 9

# Acute
# Myocardial Infarction

## PATHOPHYSIOLOGY

Coronary arteriography within 6 hours of myocardial infarction (MI) has demonstrated a thrombus occluding the infarct-related coronary artery in approximately 85% of cases(1). Although this thrombotic occlusion may be the result of multiple interacting factors(2) (hemorrhage into a plaque, platelet aggregation with release of vasoconstrictive substances, and/or coronary spasm), it occurs in the setting of significant underlying coronary atherosclerosis in more than 90% of cases. The remaining small number of infarctions without coronary atherosclerosis has been attributed to coronary embolism, isolated coronary spasm, arteritis, trauma, congenital abnormalities, and hematologic disorders(3).

## CLINICAL PRESENTATION

### Symptoms

The major symptom of an acute myocardial infarction (AMI) is **chest pain**, classically described as a substernal squeezing or pressure sensation, often radiating into the neck or down the arms (usually the left), lasting 15-30 min or longer. At times the pain may be atypical and described as burning, dull-aching, or sharp. It may even be localized just to the arms or neck without associated chest pain. **Other symptoms may include** shortness of breath, weakness, diaphoresis, and nausea.

Two important findings from the Framingham study(4) deserve mention: 1) only 23% of first MIs were preceded by a history of angina; and 2) one out of every five MIs was clinically silent or unrecognized, i.e., the pain was atypical in nature or other complaints, such as fatigue or shortness of breath, predominated so that the possibility of an MI was not considered. **Painless MI** is more frequent in diabetic patients and in the elderly. Certainly, some patients tend to deny or minimize their symptoms leading to diagnostic difficulties.

## Signs

Physical findings in patients with AMI vary; however, some generalizations can be made, assuming that pulmonary edema and/or cardiogenic shock is not present:

1. **Appearance.** Normal to diaphoretic, pale, anxious.

2. **Vital Signs.** Mild to moderate increase in heart rate (bradyarrhythmias commonly occur with inferior MI); blood pressure is usually elevated; respirations may be increased. Fever is common and rarely exceeds $103^{\circ}$ F or persists beyond the 8th day post-MI.

3. **Lungs.** If left ventricular (LV) dysfunction is present, rales or overt pulmonary edema may be seen. Otherwise, the lungs are clear.

4. **Heart.** S1 is usually of normal intensity but may be soft. New systolic murmurs may be heard (see below). The apical impulse may become diffuse and paradoxical (outward during systole). Paradoxical splitting of S2 may be heard due to a prolonged LV ejection time. An S4 is commonly noted and occasionally a soft S3 is present[5] (due to ischemia-induced decrease in ventricular compliance).

A **friction rub** secondary to pericarditis (usually associated with a transmural MI) may be heard. A friction rub usually consists of two or three components (systolic, early and late diastolic) and may occur within hours of acute infarction. Generally, the rub is intermittent, transient, lasts hours to days, and can be heard in almost every patient with a transmural MI if listened for. **New systolic murmurs**[6] may occur and should be listened for carefully and documented accurately. Such murmurs are due to:

1. **Mitral regurgitation secondary to transient ischemia or infarction of the base of the papillary muscle** leading to papillary muscle dysfunction. This murmur can be early, mid, late,or holosystolic in character. Pulmonary edema is a rare complication.

2. **Mitral regurgitation secondary to papillary muscle rupture,** as opposed to the murmur of papillary muscle dysfunction described above, is always hemodynamically significant and generally leads to pulmonary edema (see section on complications).

3. **Ventricular septal defect secondary to rupture of the septum** (see section on Complications of AMI--Recognition and Management).

DIAGNOSTIC TESTS(7)

## Electrocardiogram

The electrocardiographic diagnosis of an AMI(8) depends upon **serial ECG tracings** since it is not uncommon in the first few hours of an infarction to have absent or indeterminant ECG findings. Moreover, a classical history and a high index of suspicion should not be influenced by the initial lack of ECG findings. Patients with previous bundle branch block or artificially paced rhythms present difficulties in electrocardiographic diagnosis due to secondary ST-T wave changes, but serial tracings may demonstrate changes.

Acute inferior, anterior, or lateral **transmural myocardial ischemic injury is associated with ST segment elevation**, i.e., a "subepicardial injury pattern," in those leads which reflect the affected area of the heart (see Chapter 1). The T wave in those leads initially is upright, may be very tall or peaked, and subsequently inverts as **Q waves develop with infarction/necrosis.**

A **posterior transmural MI** is represented by an ST segment vector which is directly posterior and reflected as **ST segment depression** on the ECG in leads V1 and V2. The T wave is initially inverted, but usually becomes upright (positive) in these leads as a 40-msec R wave develops, representing unopposed anterior depolarization.

The **T waves** in a so-called **nontransmural (NTMI) or subendocardial myocardial infarction** become symmetrically inverted within minutes to hours after the acute event and remain inverted for at least 24 to 48 hours. They may remain inverted indefinitely but, on many occasions, eventually return to normal. The **ST segment** may be depressed within minutes to hours of the acute event and usually returns to baseline after several days. Q waves do not develop and there is no distinct change in the R wave. The persistence of the above changes for more than 24 hours distinguishes a NTMI from a prolonged ischemic episode without infarction.

## Cardiac Enzymes

The serum enzymes used most frequently to diagnose acute myocardial infarction are **creatine kinase (CK), serum glutamic oxaloacetic transaminase (SGOT), and lactic dehydrogenase (LDH)**(9,10). Each enzyme demonstrates a characteristic pattern of rise and fall in myocardial infarction which, when followed serially, greatly aids in the diagnosis of an AMI. A brief description of each enzyme and a table of characteristic changes in an AMI follow:

1. **CK.** Sometimes referred to as "CPK," this enzyme is released with any muscle injury or trauma. **The specificity of an elevated CK improves by measuring the CK isoenzyme, CK-MB.** This isoenzyme is found in high concentration in cardiac muscle as opposed to skeletal muscle and is elevated with myocardial injury. Elevation does not occur with other muscle injuries unless significant skeletal muscle destruction has occurred, i.e., rhabdomyolysis, polymyositis, etc.

   The sensitivity of CK-MB detection varies with the isoenzyme assay technique used. Abnormal absolute values (usually >5 IU/L) may vary from institution to institution. In addition, it has been suggested that the percentage of CK as CK-MB might improve diagnostic sensitivity (>5% CK-MB/total CK abnormal). The house officer should be familiar with his/her institutional normal CK and CK-MB values.

2. **SGOT.** This enzyme is relatively nonspecific, being found in numerous tissues of the body.

3. **LDH.** Total serum LDH is of very low specificity for an AMI since it is present in nearly every tissue in the body. However, LDH is composed of **five isoenzymes** of which LDH1 and LDH2 are found primarily in cardiac muscle. The normal LDH1:LDH2 ratio is $\leq 1.0$. Isoenzyme determination by electrophoresis **may be of value in diagnosis of AMI if the patient presents more than 24 hours** after the acute ischemic event and the LDH1:LDH2 ratio increases.

Table 9.1
Enzyme Course in Acute MI

| Enzyme | Earliest Rise | Peak | Normalize |
|--------|---------------|------|-----------|
| CK | 6 hours | 24–30 hours | 3–4 days |
| CK-MB | 4–6 hours | 18–24 hours | 36–48 hours |
| SGOT | 8–12 hours | 36–48 hours | 3–5 days |
| LDH | 12–24 hours | 2–4 days | 7–10 days |

**Radionuclide Scanning**

In the majority of AMIs, the clinical history, ECG, and pattern of enzyme changes will establish the diagnosis without difficulty, and radionuclide scanning will add little useful information. However, in certain situations where the clinical history, ECG, and/or enzyme pattern is confusing or not available, a properly timed radionuclide scan can be helpful in establishing the diagnosis. Two techniques utilizing either technetium pyrophosphate or thallium-201 are available (see Chapter 5).

**Technetium pyrophosphate,** a calcium-avid radioisotope, is deposited in irreversibly ischemic myocardial tissue and yields a "hot spot" on nuclear imaging.  The scintigram first becomes positive within 10 to 12 hours after an acute infarction, but becomes increasingly more positive 24 to 72 hours post-MI.  A 3+ diffuse or localized uptake (uptake equivalent to bone) is very suggestive of a recent MI.  The diagnostic **specificity** of pyrophosphate scanning is highest in patients with no previous infarction.  Diagnostic **sensitivity** in transmural infarction is 84-95% if local deposition is seen.  In subendocardial infarction, 32% of patients demonstrate a localized pattern, 19% demonstrate a diffuse pattern, and 50% have no discernible uptake, i.e., a negative scan (11).

**Thallium-201** exchanges with potassium in normal cells and therefore yields a myocardial "cold spot" in the presence of an old or new myocardial infarction or an area of relative ischemia.  Thus, thallium scintigrams have **poor specificity** for AMI because reduced uptake can be due to ischemia, old or new infarction, or a combination of these. Assuming that no previous infarctions have occurred, the thallium scan will be very sensitive during the first 24 hours in an AMI.  Due to the lack of ready availability of thallium, the cumbersome machinery involved, and the fact that each thallium injection is equivalent in radiation dosage to an intravenous pyelogram, thallium-201 is usually not used routinely to diagnose an AMI.

## PROGNOSTIC CONSIDERATIONS

### Infarct Size

The amount of damaged myocardium and resultant left ventricular dysfunction is the principal determinant of outcome following MI(12). Infarct size varies from minimal loss of myocardial muscle mass (less than 5% in-hospital mortality) to loss of approximately 40% of the LV muscle mass and resultant cardiogenic shock (in-hospital mortality often >80%). **No perfect method of infarct size assessment is available**(13); however, clinicians make general estimates based on clinical status, CK values, ECGs, nuclear ventriculography, two-dimensional echocardiography, and abnormalities during invasive hemodynamic monitoring(14). **Limiting infarct size** has been attempted using agents that decrease the oxygen demands of the myocardium (nitroglycerin, beta blockers, calcium blockers, etc.) and/or by increasing supply (thrombolytic therapy, angioplasty, and coronary bypass surgery)(15).  Studies assessing benefit of interventions designed to limit infarct size must be interpreted cautiously in view of the imprecise methods of quantitation. Research techniques utilizing positron emission tomography and magnetic resonance imaging (MRI) may prove to be of value(16).

## Infarct Site

The site of the infarct is an important variable in determining outcome. **Anterior MIs** generally result from occlusion of the left anterior descending coronary artery. They tend to be larger infarcts and therefore are associated with a higher mortality. These infarcts are more prone to expansion, rupture, mural thrombus, and aneurysm formation. Occlusion of the circumflex coronary artery results in **lateral infarction.** When the circumflex is a dominant artery (10% of cases) the infarct may involve the posterior and inferior walls(3).

Right coronary artery occlusion may result in **inferior** or **inferoposterior infarction.** Although right coronary occlusion usually causes less loss of critical myocardium than obstruction of the left anterior descending branch, the spectrum of clinical presentation varies widely from a "benign" event to major hemodynamic consequences (right ventricular infarction, rupture of the posteromedial papillary muscle), and significant arrhythmias (bradycardia, heart block, and ventricular fibrillation).

## Coexistent Coronary Artery Disease

Another factor affecting outcome of myocardial infarction is the presence of coexistent coronary artery disease in vessels supplying noninfarcted myocardium. Seventy-five percent of AMI patients have at least two major vessels with critical lesions and 50% have triple vessel disease(3). It thus follows that angina may develop early after infarct (within 7 to 10 days) in approximately 25% of acute MI patients and is often associated with a poor prognosis. Patients with angina from "ischemia at a distance" (outside the zone of infarct) are now recognized as having a high mortality at 6 months (75%)(17).

### ACUTE INTERVENTION IN AMI-REPERFUSION

Until recently, treatment of AMI was largely expectant or prophylactic in character or directed toward the management of complications as discussed later. Limitation of the size of infarction is the goal of the acute interventions which are now being used with increasing frequency. Early use of thrombolytic therapy, emergency percutaneous transluminal coronary angioplasty, and emergency coronary bypass surgery have all been used at various centers with a variable success rate. No intervention has been conclusively proven to result in myocardial salvage or reduce mortality despite widespread enthusiasm for these techniques.

## Thrombolytic Therapy

Both intravenous and intracoronary thombolytic therapy have been shown to be successful in relieving pain and restoring flow in the infarct related coronary artery in the majority of patients(18). These benefits have to be weighed against the expense, risks of potential bleeding problems, creation of an unstable state with a subtotal lesion in a recanalized artery, potential extension of infarction, arrhythmias, and allergic reactions.

Coronary angiography and administration of **intracoronary streptokinase** can be carried out safely and successful clot lysis with restoration of flow can be achieved in approximately 70 to 80% of patients presenting within the first 6 hours of onset of symptoms(18).  It is often difficult to determine to what degree there has been myocardial salvage(19,20); this is a problem, in part, because of the limited abilities of invasive and noninvasive assessments of wall motion and ventricular function.

**Intravenous streptokinase**(21) is less successful in achieving recanalization but has the attractive advantage of ease of administration which would permit more widespread early use. With successful reperfusion, one usually sees an accelerated electrocardiographic course and rapid acceleration of CK appearance.

Despite the enthusiasm for thrombolysis in acute MI, there are limited data to indicate that myocardium in jeopardy is salvaged or that long-term outcome is improved.

A new fibrin-specific thrombolytic agent, **tissue-type plasminogen activator** (t-PA), has been developed and is currently undergoing clinical trials. Preliminary results suggest that intravenous t-PA is as effective as intracoronary streptokinase in achieving recanalization of acutely occluded coronary arteries without the time, risk, and specialized equipment and personnel required for emergent coronary arteriography(22).  The occurrence of bleeding complications was similar to that seen in patients receiving streptokinase.

## Percutaneous Transluminal Coronary Angioplasty (PTCA)

PTCA has been used by a number of centers as initial therapy of AMI (23,24).  Not all patients are candidates for this therapy but many could benefit from urgent recanalization. Advantages over thrombolytic therapy include a shorter total time in the catheterization laboratory, definitive management of the underlying stenosis, and no effect on systemic coagulation.  Dissection of the balloon-dilated coronary artery is a common occurrence with uncertain long-term implications. A coronary bypass surgical team should be available when the procedure is performed.

## Emergency Bypass Surgery

Emergency coronary bypass surgery has the potential value of myocardial salvage if difficult logistics can be handled within the first 4 hours of myocardial infarction.  Surgery should be considered in patients whose coronary anatomy has been previously assessed with angiography and who develop ischemia while in the hospital awaiting surgery or in those who develop the onset of myocardial infarction while undergoing routine angiography or coronary angioplasty. Bypass of diseased but noninfarct-related arteries at the time of surgery could have additional value. However, the usual delay in clinical presentation of the patient who develops MI out of the hospital and the time required for clinical evaluation, angiography, assembling the surgical team, and placing the patient on cardiopulmonary bypass will generally preclude this intervention in most patients.

### Reperfusion Injury

Reperfusion injury occurs in myocardium which is perfused with blood following as little as 1 hour of total occlusion(25). The damage resulting from reperfusion is biochemically complex and largely due to free radical-mediated injury to membrane phospholipids (lipid peroxidation). Experimental approaches to avoid this paradox are being studied and include reperfusion with blood-free solutions and free radical scavengers.

### COMPLICATIONS OF AMI-RECOGNITION AND MANAGEMENT CARDIAC RHYTHM DISTURBANCES

Prompt recognition and treatment of arrhythmias is important in order to minimize their deleterious hemodynamic effects (reduced cardiac output and increased myocardial oxygen demand--$MVO_2$-- and their tendency to lead to more serious electrical instability.

### Supraventricular Arrhythmias:

Excluding sinus tachycardia and sinus bradycardia, there is an overall 24 to 40% incidence of supraventricular arrhythmias in the setting of AMI(26).

1.  **Sinus Tachycardia.** This condition is detrimental in the setting of myocardial ischemia due to the increase in $MVO_2$ in the presence of fixed blood supply. With adequate pain control, appropriate sedation, no fever, and no clinical evidence of LV failure, sinus rates of >110 may need investigation with a pulmonary artery flotation catheter to determine the underlying etiology: hypovolemia, subclinical LV failure, or hyperadrenergic state. **Therapy consists of treating the underlying abnormality.** Beta blockers (e.g., propranolol, 0.05-0.1 mg/kg IV total dose administered over 30 min) may be used for the control of sinus tachycardia in isolated hyperadrenergic states (normal PCWP, increased cardiac output, increased heart rate). Digoxin should not be used to treat sinus tachycardia in the absence of LV failure. Decreased preload (low PCWP) can be treated with judicious volume

challenge using normal saline or a colloid solution.

2. **Sinus Bradycardia.** Bradycardia may be transient or persistent and may be associated with hypotension. The combination of hypotension and bradycardia usually represents a vasovagal reaction (Bezold-Jarisch reflex) and is a common occurrence in acute inferior MI. Therapy is not required unless the patient is symptomatic or the bradyarrhythmia is accompanied by premature ventricular contractions (PVCs) or escape rhythms. **Atropine (0.5 mg to 2.0 mg) is the drug of choice for treatment of symptomatic or hemodynamically compromising bradycardia-hypotension**(27). If atropine is ineffective or frequently required, then an atrial or ventricular temporary pacemaker is indicated.

3. **Premature atrial Contractions (15–40% Incidence).** These are usually of no hemodynamic or prognostic significance, except that sustained episodes of supraventricular tachycardia (SVT) may be initiated (see below). Treatment with quinidine or procainamide is indicated for recurrent SVT prophylaxis and/or frequent premature atrial contractions (>10/min).

4. **Paroxysmal Supraventricular Tachycardia (2–7% Incidence).** There are two basic types: 1) **Re-entrant supraventricular tachycardia (R-SVT),** and 2) **automatic atrial tachycardia (AAT)** (see Chapter 2). Therapy varies for the two types.

   **R-SVT.** Vagal maneuvers, such as carotid sinus massage, may break the rhythm; parasympathomimetic or adrenergic drugs are contraindicated. Cardioversion (50 watt/sec) is indicated if there is evidence of hemodynamic compromise. Recurrent episodes can be treated with digoxin, quinidine/procainamide, verapamil, or beta-blocking drugs.

   **AAT.** Vagal maneuvers and atrial pacing are not effective in AAT. Suppression of automaticity is necessary with quinidine or procainamide. Sympathomimetic drugs should be discontinued.

5. **Atrial Fibrillation (10% Incidence).** In the setting of an acute MI, this rhythm is usually encountered in congestive heart failure (CHF), atrial infarction, or pericarditis. Ninety percent of episodes of atrial fibrillation occur within the first 48 hours and usually last less than 24 hours. Recurrence is common. DC synchronized countershock (100–400 W/sec) should be used to treat acute episodes associated with hypoperfusion or prolonged episodes not responsive to pharmacologic management. If first attempts at electrical cardioversion are not successful, procainamide (500-1000 mg IV over 20-30 min) can be given and synchronized countershock attempted again. Medical management would include the use of IV digoxin, verapamil, and/or a beta blocker in patients without

contraindications to use of these drugs (see Chapter 2). Following electrical or chemical cardioversion, "suppressive" pharmacologic agents should be initiated or continued.

6. **Atrial Flutter (5% Incidence).** This unstable rhythm may be either transient (spontaneous conversion to normal sinus rhythm [NSR] or atrial fibrillation) or sustained. Cardioversion (50 W/sec) is the treatment of choice for sustained episodes. If recurrent, the use of rapid (overdrive) atrial pacing to break the rhythm may be helpful.

7. **Junctional Tachycardia (5-10% Incidence).** This rhythm disturbance is caused by enhanced automaticity of the junctional pacemaker and is usually due to atrioventricular (AV) node ischemia or drugs, especially digoxin at toxic concentrations. It is usually self-limited and treatment is not indicated unless loss of atrial contraction causes hemodynamic deterioration or ischemia. It can be treated with lidocaine, procainamide, or atrial overdrive pacing.

**Ventricular Arrhythmias:**

**Prophylactic Antiarrhythmic Therapy(28).** It is our policy that most patients with acute or possible acute infarction be given prophylactic lidocaine, rather than waiting for warning arrhythmias to develop because:

1. Warning arrhythmias are not reliable predictors of primary ventricular fibrillation (PVF). Twenty-five to 50% of patients who develop PVF in the Coronary Care Unit (CCU) have no warning arrhythmias.

2. Less than half of all warning arrhythmias are detected by the CCU staff.

Prophylactic lidocaine has been shown to be effective in reducing the incidence of PVF(28). The **loading dose** is 200 mg divided into two doses, given 20 minutes apart, or 75 mg initially and 50-mg boluses at 5-min intervals to a total dose of 225 mg(29). A **constant infusion** (with an infusion pump) of 2 mg/min should be started with the first dose. The maximum infusion rate is 4 mg/min. The **loading dose and infusion rate should be reduced** by half in the presence of CHF, shock, liver disease, or a patient 70 years of age or older. The infusion can be stopped (not tapered) at 36 hours in the absence of ventricular arrhythmias. If ventricular ectopy develops with cessation of the infusion, lidocaine should be restarted and continued for another 24-36 hours. If complex ventricular ectopy, i.e., multiform, runs or pairs, or frequent PVCs (>6/min), develop when the infusion is stopped, chronic oral antiarrhythmics may be necessary.

1. **Premature Ventricular Contractions.** Almost all patients will have PVCs during the acute phase of MI. Complete or nearly complete

suppression of ventricular ectopy in the acute phase of an infarction is the goal of therapy. If lidocaine is not effective consider:

A. **Procainamide.** Administer 100 mg every 5 min until ectopy is controlled or a 1-gm total dose is given. For malignant life-threatening arrhythmias, higher loading doses may be required (i.e., 2 gms) and are usually tolerated without difficulty. **Monitor BP and EKG closely** since hypotension and conduction disturbances (prolonged QRS duration and QT interval) can occur if dose is given too rapidly. After loading is completed, a constant infusion at 2-3 mg/min should be started, with a maximum rate of 4 mg/min. A bolus of 50-75 mg of procainamide should be employed whenever the infusion rate is increased.

B. **Bretylium.** Five-10 mg/kg can be administered IV over 10 min, followed by a constant infusion of a rate of 1-2 mg/min. After an initial increase in blood pressure, hypotension may occur due to the blocking of the efferent limb of the baroreceptor reflex. Initial sinus tachycardia may be due to catecholamine release. Bretylium should not be used in patients with a fixed cardiac output, e.g., severe aortic stenosis. Postural hypotension is a common complication.

C. A combination of procainamide and lidocaine may be used but can result in neurotoxicity (altered mental status, seizures) since the two drugs have additive central nervous system (CNS) effects; combined infusion rate should not exceed 5 mg/min.

2. **Ventricular Tachycardia.** This rhythm is defined as $\geq$ 3 consecutive PVCs at a rate of 120/min or greater. Therapy is dictated by the clinical status of the patient. If transient or sustained without clinical evidence of hypoperfusion, intravenous lidocaine may be used (see above). Synchronized countershock at 50-400 W/sec should be employed if the rhythm is sustained and associated with hemodynamic deterioration.

3. **Accelerated Idioventricular Rhythm (8-23% Incidence).** This rhythm may be the result of enhanced automaticity of an ectopic ventricular pacemaker or the result of variable exit block of a focus of ventricular tachycardia. The wide ectopic QRS complexes occur at regular intervals, resulting in atrioventricular dissociation when the prevailing supraventricular rhythm slows below the intrinsic rate of the idioventricular pacemaker (60-90/min). It is usually benign and does not result in PVF(30). Close monitoring for 24 hours is advisable because of rare association with ventricular tachycardia. If the rhythm is not hemodynamically tolerated, suppression with lidocaine, procainamide, or atropine (by increasing the sinus rate) can be employed. Overdrive atrial pacing is also effective. Treatment is infrequently necessary.

## AV BLOCK AND VENTRICULAR CONDUCTION DISTURBANCES

The incidence of progression to high-degree AV block, without previous ECG evidence of conduction disturbance, is approximately 6%. The onset of complete heart block (CHB) is different, depending on the site of infarction:

**Inferior MI.**   Complete heart block is the result of increased vagal tone or ischemia of the AV node. CHB rarely occurs suddenly. Progression from first-degree block to various degrees of second degree AV block usually precedes CHB. During CHB, the heart rate is generally 50 beats/min, and QRS is commonly narrow. Treatment ranges from observation in the stable patient to using IV atropine in the hemodynamically unstable patient (dosage of 0.5 mg IV up to 2 mg IV).

**Anterior MI.**   Caused by ischemia or infarction of the His bundle or both bundle branches, CHB frequently develops suddenly and results in wide, bizarre QRS complexes and bradycardia. Pacemaker therapy may be necessary (see Chapter 17 for recommendations regarding prophylactic pacemaker insertion in the face of acute myocardial infarction). Any patient who develops permanent or transient high-degree AV block associated with bundle branch block during an MI should have a permanent pacemaker implanted.

## PERSISTENT AND RECURRENT ISCHEMIC CHEST PAIN

Recurrent chest pain during and after the first 24 hours is not unusual and is often relieved with nitrates alone. Nitroglycerin should be used in small doses (0.4 mg sublingual) in normotensive patients. If chest pain persists or recurs, consider(31):

1. A combination of sublingual nitroglycerin tablets and parenteral morphine (in incremental 2-mg IV doses). Adequate sedation is usually achieved with morphine.

2. If the pain persists or recurs and hypotension is not present, start topical nitroglycerin ointment at 1/2 inch every 4 hours with a rapid stepwise increase to 2 inches every 4 hours if necessary.

3. If the above are ineffective, start **IV nitroglycerin**--40 mg in 250 cc of 5% dextrose in water at 5 cc/hour. IV nitroglycerin can be safely administered to hemodynamically stable patients without pulmonary artery (PA) pressure monitoring. Usual range of nitroglycerin needed for pain control is 0.7 to 2.0 mu/kg/min. In invasively monitored patients, fluids should be administered if PCWP falls below 15 mm Hg and is associated with a significant drop in blood pressure or cardiac output. If clinical evidence of hypoperfusion occurs in a patient without PA pressure monitoring in the low dose range, fluids should be given judiciously and a PA catheter

inserted.  IV nitroglycerin is an arterial vasodilator as well as a venodilator; therefore, attempts to maintain blood pressure by volume challenge may not always be successful.  The rationale of IV nitroglycerin therapy is reduction of $MVO_2$, coronary vasodilation, promotion of collateral supply, and reversal of any coronary spasm(32).

4.  If pain recurs or persists despite maximal IV nitroglycerin, **IV propranolol** or metoprolol may be used if PCWP is less than 18 and cardiac index is greater than 2.4 L/min/$M^2$.  Invasive pressure monitoring is recommended.  Propranolol can be given in 1-mg doses every 10-15 minutes to a total dose of 0.05-0.1 mg/kg.  Metoprolol can be given in 5 mg boluses at 2 minute intervals to a total dose of 15 mg.  In the setting of an AMI, beta blocking agents may affect the myocardium unpredictably and their use must be monitored closely.  If acutely effective and tolerated, beta blockers can then be given orally— propranolol 20-80 mg q6h or metoprolol 50-100 mg q12h.

5.  **Calcium channel blockers** may be used in addition to, or in place of, beta blockers for pain control.  There are three currently available calcium channel blockers in the United States:

   A.  **Nifedipine** has the most potent vasodilator and antihypertensive effects of the three.  It has essentially no negative inotropic effect and is the calcium channel blocker of choice for use in patients with chest pain and hypertension or congestive heart failure.  The usual dosage range is from 10 mg P.O. t.i.d. to 30 mg P.O. q.i.d.

   B.  **Verapamil** is the strongest negative inotrope of the calcium channel blockers.  It also has the most potent blocking effects on the AV node as well as some negative chronotropic effect on the sinoatrial (SA) node.  It is the calcium channel blocker of choice for use in patients with chest pain and supraventricular tachycardias.  Its use is contraindicated in patients with congestive heart failure and it should be used cautiously in patients who are receiving beta blocking drugs.  The usual dosage range is from 80 mg P.O. t.i.d. to 120 mg P.O. q.i.d.  It is the only currently available calcium-blocker in parenteral (IV) form.  Acute IV use should be limited to 5-15 mg given in divided doses over 15-30 min.

   C.  **Diltiazem** is the most recent of the calcium channel-blocking agents available in the United States.  Its effects on AV nodal conduction and LV performance are intermediate between those of nifedipine and verapamil.  It has the least antihypertensive effect of the three drugs.  The usual dosage range is from 60 mg P.O. t.i.d. to 120 mg P.O. q.i.d.

If a low BP or CI or a high PCWP prohibit the use of beta blockers or calcium channel blockers or they are not effective, intra-aortic balloon pumping (IABP) (see below) and continued IV nitroglycerin and propranolol may result in pain relief.

Coronary arteriography and coronary revascularization or PTCA should be considered if the above measures fail to control symptoms.

## HEMODYNAMIC DECOMPENSATION DUE TO PUMP FAILURE

An acute myocardial infarction almost always causes some degree of acute LV dysfunction. Whether this dysfunction becomes clinically apparent or important depends on the amount of myocardium damaged; a loss of myocardium greater than 40% generally leads to cardiogenic shock. Several classifications have been developed which correlate LV dysfunction during an AMI to in-hospital mortality. The **Killip Classification**(33) is one of the most frequently quoted and is based entirely on clinical findings.

**Table 9.2**

| Killip Classification | Incidence | Mortality |
|---|---|---|
| I.   No heart failure | 33% | 6% |
| II.  Mid failure (bibasilar rales) | 38% | 17% |
| III. Frank pulmonary edema | 10% | 38% |
| IV.  Cardiogenic shock (hypotension with BP of $\leq$ 90 mm Hg, peripheral vasoconstriction, oliguria, and pulmonary vascular congestion) | 19% | 81% |

A clinical, **noninvasive evaluation** of the patient with an AMI has **significant limitations** in that it will overestimate cardiac index in 25% of patients and it will underestimate PCWP in 15% of patients. Therefore, in high-risk mortality groups (Killip Classes III and IV) or in a patient with a confusing clinical picture, a PA catheter should be inserted so that therapeutic decisions can be based upon hemodynamic findings.

A classification that correlates clinical signs with invasive hemodynamic data and which is helpful in planning treatment is that of Karliner and Ross(34) shown in Table 9.3.

**Table 9.3**
**Hemodynamic Classification of the AMI Patient**

| | Clinical | Systemic Art. Pressure | Cardiac Index* | Peripheral Vasc. Res. | PCWP** |
|---|---|---|---|---|---|
| I. | Uncompl. | nl or ↓ | nl or ↑ | nl | usually ↑ |
| II. | Mild CHF | usually nl | ↓ | ↑ | ↑↑ |
| III. | Severe CHF | ↓ | ↓↓ | ↑↑ | ↑↑↑ |
| IV. | Shock: | | | | |
| | Cardiogenic | ↓↓↓ | ↓↓↓ | ↑↑↑ | ↑↑↑ |
| | Hypovolemic | ↓↓↓ | ↓↓↓ | ↑↑↑ | nl or ↓ |

*Cardiac index:   Normal (nl) = 2.5-3.6 L/min/m$^2$
                  Reduced = 2.2-2.5 L/min/m$^2$
                  Hypoperfusion = 1.8-2.2 L/min/m$^2$
                  Shock = 1.8 L/min/m$^2$

**PCWP:  Normal = 10-20 mm Hg
         Optimum with AMI = 14-18 mm Hg

**Uncomplicated.**  No specific therapy indicated.

**Mild CHF.**  Major problem is elevated PCWP.  Treatment involves reduction of preload with either diuretics or nitrates.  Remember there is a "lag period" between normalization of PCWP and disappearance of rales and radiographic resolution.

**Severe CHF.**  Elevated PCWP and significantly reduced CO are the major problems.  There are two options:  preload reduction along with diuretics or nitrates or preload and afterload reduction with nitroprusside.  The latter has the advantage of increasing CO which the former therapy does not.  Inotropic agents should be avoided to minimize $MVO_2$.

**Cardiogenic Shock.**  The major problem is a markedly reduced CI, usually <1.8 L/min/m$^2$.  If the PCWP is normal or low, fluids may increase cardiac output via Starling's Law.  Optimum PCWP is approximately 15 to 20 mm Hg in an AMI.  However, most cases usually have a very high PCWP.

The systolic pressure will primarily dictate the therapeutic approach:

1.  If the systolic pressure is greater than 100, increase cardiac index through afterload reduction with nitroprusside. If systolic pressure is less than 100, afterload reduction should be undertaken cautiously.

2.  With mild hypotension (systolic 75-90), dobutamine may improve CI and BP. Dopamine may be added to increase BP if dobutamine alone fails to do so.

3.  With significant hypotension (systolic pressure less than 75), use a pressor agent (e.g., dopamine) because rapid attainment and maintenance of an adequate BP (systolic 90-100) is of prime importance in treating cardiogenic shock. Dobutamine may be added for its effect on cardiac output but usually it will not raise the BP enough to be used without a pressor. A combination of dobutamine and dopamine may be most effective(35).

## INTRA-AORTIC BALLOON PUMP (IABP) IN CARDIOGENIC SHOCK

Ideal candidate criteria for IABP include: early in course (less than 6 hours postinfarction), younger patients, first MI, absence of any terminal disease, and no aortic insufficiency.

**Hemodynamic Effects of IABP.** Afterload is reduced and diastolic pressure is increased, thereby improving coronary perfusion pressure and cardiac output. Overall effect is to improve myocardial metabolism and decrease LV size.

**Course.** Twenty percent of AMI patients with cardiogenic shock recover to be weaned off IABP and discharged home. The remainder usually improve but continue to be IABP dependent. Heart catheterization and cardiac surgery may be beneficial. Surgery is most successful in patients with a correctible mechanical defect (i.e., ventricular septal defect (VSD), aneurysm, or ruptured papillary muscle) in addition to bypassable coronary artery obstructions.

**Complications of IABP.** There is a 15 to 30% incidence of complications(36). These include: 1) rupture of balloon; 2) emboli from balloon to kidneys or lower extremities; 3) dissection of the aorta; 4) leg ischemia resulting in neuropathy, myopathy, or amputation; 5) groin infections; 6) thrombocytopenia and anemia; and 7) leg claudication. Embolic phenomena are markedly decreased by the use of anticoagulation with heparin during IABP therapy.

## RIGHT VENTRICULAR INFARCTION

This complication is almost exclusively associated with acute inferior infarction. Nineteen to 43% of inferior infarctions are complicated by right ventricular (RV) involvement, but only 3 to 8% of these have clinical findings suggestive of right ventricular dysfunction, such as neck vein distention or arterial hypotension(37). The syndrome of hypotension and low cardiac output associated with a right ventricular infarction is attributed to the inability of the infarcted right ventricle to maintain adequate left ventricular filling.

### Confirm the Diagnosis by:

1. **ECG.**  An ECG sign of RV infarct is the presence of ST elevation in the right precordial leads, especially V4R(38).

2. **Swan-Ganz Catheter.**  Elevated mean right atrial pressures (12-20 mm Hg) which is equal to or greater than the PCWP(39).

3. **Gated Cardiac Blood Pool Scan.**  Poor right ventricular function(40).

Therapy includes:  1) plasma expanders to increase the pressure gradient in the right heart, favoring increased passive flow through the lungs to the left heart (follow PCWP as a guide to fluid therapy), and 2) afterload reduction of the left heart to increase cardiac output and decrease left atrial pressure, encouraging passive filling from the right heart(41).

Cardiogenic shock due to predominant RV dysfunction is uncommon; however, this is an important entity to recognize because it represents a treatable subset of cardiogenic shock with a survival of better than 50% compared to 10-15% survival in shock due to anterior LV wall infarction(37).

## COMPLICATIONS OF AMI SECONDARY TO MECHANICAL DEFECTS

### Mechanical Defects Causing Decompensation:

1. **Ruptured Papillary Muscle**(42).

   - **Clinical Picture.**  Sudden appearance of an apical systolic murmur associated with abrupt clinical LV failure.  Course may be less severe if only papillary head and not the entire body of the muscle is ruptured.

   - **Incidence.**  Incidence is 1 to 5% among patients dying of an acute myocardial infarction.  Occurs 2 to 10 days post-MI, primarily involves the posterior side of the papillary muscle, and is associated with inferior-posterior MI.

- **Mortality.**  Seventy percent within 24 hours; 90% within two weeks.

- **Diagnosis.**  Large V waves on PCWP tracing (see Figure 11.3B). Two-dimensional echocardiogram may show the ruptured papillary muscle.  Doppler echocardiography will demonstrate severe mitral regurgitation.

- **Therapy.**

  a) Afterload reduction with nitroprusside; if ineffective, consider IABP.

  b) If stabilized medically, surgery in weeks to months.  If unstable and in need of IABP, cardiac catheterization is indicated and possibly immediate surgery.

2. **Ventricular Septal Rupture**(42).

   - **Clinical Picture.**  Very similar to ruptured papillary muscle. Sudden onset of harsh systolic murmur along the left sternal border associated with hemodynamic deterioration.

   - **Incidence.**  Incidence is 0.5 to 1% accounting for approximately 2% of deaths following an infarction.  Usually associated with an anteroseptal infarction occurring 9 to 10 days postinfarction. Rupture commonly involves the apical anterior muscular septum.

   - **Mortality.**  Twenty-four percent within 24 hours; 87% within 2 months.

   - **Diagnosis.**  Oxygen saturation step-up in the pulmonary artery as compared to right atrium in blood samples drawn from Swan-Ganz catheter.  Echocardiography may demonstrate the defect in the interventricular septum.  Doppler echocardiography will show flow from left to right across the defect.

   - **Therapy.**  Same as for ruptured papillary muscle.

3. **Cardiac Rupture**(43).

   - **Clinical Picture.**  Sudden chest pain followed immediately by hypotension, electromechanical dissociation, and death.  Symptoms of cardiac tamponade may develop prior to death.

   - **Incidence.**  Reported to occur in up to 24% of fatal AMIs.  More common than papillary muscle or ventricular septal rupture. Fifty percent of cases occur within 5 days postinfarction and 90% within 2 weeks.  More common in females.

   - **High-Risk Patients.**  First infarction, sustained hypertension after myocardial infarction, and patients over 80 years of age.

More common in those undergoing infarct expansion.

- **Therapy.** Volume replacement, repeated pericardiocentesis, open-chest resuscitation if needed, and immediate transfer to operating room. Mortality is 95%.

## EMBOLIC COMPLICATIONS OF AMI

### Pulmonary Embolism:

With the advent of early ambulation in patients with AMI, incidence of pulmonary embolism has seemingly decreased. Predisposing factors include: LV failure, arrhythmias, old age, obesity, and varicose veins. Low dose heparin (5,000 units subcutaneously b.i.d.) markedly reduces the incidence of DVT in AMI patients and should, therefore, reduce the incidence of pulmonary emboli.

### Arterial Embolism:

Older studies (prior to 1973) have quoted a 2.5 to 4.9% incidence of arterial emboli to the brain, kidneys, or limbs, supposedly from intraventricular mural thrombus overlying the infarction. There are no current figures; clinically, the incidence seems less. Recommendations regarding the use of prophylactic anticoagulation therapy vary among institutions. Therapeutic recommendations include anticoagulation in patients with echo or nuclear scan documented new ventricular aneurysms or mural clots(44).

## HYPERTENSION

Hypertension is not uncommon in the early phase of an acute myocardial infarction. It has many possible causes, including underlying essential hypertension, CHF, or elevated catecholamines secondary to chest pain or anxiety. Hypertension causes an increase in intraventricular pressure which results in an increased $MVO_2$ via LaPlace's Law. This may worsen ischemia and even cause extension of the MI. If the patient is seen early in the infarction period (less than 6 hours after the onset of pain) or has evidence of ongoing ischemia (recurrent chest pain), cautious but aggressive management of hypertension is recommended in hopes of modifying infarct size.

1.  Attempt to adequately control chest pain with nitrates and/or morphine.

2.  Sedation if patient is anxious.

3.  If BP remains elevated, continue the use of nitrates and cautiously use low doses of diuretics.

4.  If the BP remains significantly elevated, the use of IV medication is warranted. A Swan-Ganz catheter is suggested to monitor left ventricular filling pressures. With mild cases, IV nitroglycerin

is recommended, but with a markedly elevated BP, nitroprusside should be given at a starting dose of 0.5 to 1.0 mu/kg/min. An arterial line is recommended when using nitroprusside.

**Table 9.4**
**Summary of Indications for Balloon-Tipped Thermodilution Catheter in AMI**

1. Killip Class III or IV.

2. Hypotension.

3. Hypertension requiring intravenous antihypertensive drugs.

4. Persistent or recurrent chest pain.

5. Differentiation of postinfarct VSD from papillary muscle rupture.

## INFARCT EXPANSION

Cardiac dilatation after MI is not clearly understood but does portend a poor prognosis(45,46). Transmural infarction is more prone to dilatation whereas nontransmural infarct patients tend to be spared this phenomenon. Usually the infarct segment involves more than 10% of the left ventricle although there is not a clear correlation between infarct size and extent of expansion.

## ANEURYSM

An aneurysm is defined as a convex protrusion of the full thickness of the left ventricular wall scar. Clinical complications which bring this entity to attention are congestive heart failure, malignant arrhythmias,and systemic emboli. Pathologic distinction between 2 types of aneuryisms has been made based on the endocardial pathology(47). A type 1 aneurysm has extensive endocardial fibroelastosis which appears as dense white collagen layering the infarct site. This type is devoid of thrombus, but is often associated with malignant ventricular arrhythmias. Fibroelastosis generally occurs after 1 year and is often the time of onset of ventricular tachycardia. The understanding of this pathology has led to recent advances in endocardial stripping procedures in combination with aneurysmectomy in patients having surgery for intractable arrhythmias. A type 2 aneurysm contains little fibroelastosis but frequently has abundant mural thrombus. Both types can result in congestive heart failure.

## MURAL THROMBUS

Stasis of flow and endocardial injury are the common factors in forming a left ventricular thrombus. This entity generally occurs in transmural anterior infarcts with akinetic or dyskinetic segments. Two-dimensional echocardiography is valuable in diagnosing this condition. Anticoagulation has not been proven effective in preventing embolization but its use seems prudent in many cases(44).

## SUBENDOCARDIAL MI

Definition:

A subendocardial MI is characterized by typical chest pain, serum enzyme elevation, and persistent (greater than 48 hours) new T wave inversion, ST segment depression, or both, in the absence of new pathologic Q waves(48).

Pathophysiology:

Nontransmural infarcts are generally smaller than transmural infarcts because an epicardial rim of myocardium is preserved. This preserved area is probably the result of collateral flow which often reflects more severe long-standing coronary artery disease (CAD). The viable tissue remaining after subendocardial MI is particularly prone to recurrent ischemia and its electrical consequences(49).

Clinical Course:

In the Mayo Clinic Study, 30% of patients with subendocardial MIs developed stable angina and 46% developed unstable angina within 1 year of the initial event. Transmural infarct developed in 21% of the medically treated group. Angiographic studies in these patients showed a narrowing of greater than 75% in at least one vessel in all patients; 60% of these patients had double- or triple-vessel disease(48).

Other studies have shown that there is no significant difference in mortality in comparing transmural and subendocardial MIs, and that patients with subendocardial MI are more prone to sudden cardiac death(50).

Implications:

Although often misconstrued as a "benign" event, subendocardial MI is often the forerunner of serious problems. Medical therapy with nitrates, beta blockers,and calcium blockers are used when feasible and appropriate patients should be studied early in the catheterization laboratory and considered for revascularization with angioplasty or coronary bypass surgery.

## REINFARCTION

Recurrent chest pain and sudden deterioration of functional status, as well as secondary elevation of plasma CPK-MB, are the clues that reinfarction has occurred. Eighty-five percent of reinfarctions occur during the initial hospitalization (between the third and tenth hospital day)(51). The overall incidence is 25% of cases, with an incidence of 10% in transmural MIs, and 42% in subendocardial MIs. Along with recurrent chest pain and the clinical setting of subendocardial MI, other predictors of extension of MI are female gender and obesity. Early reinfarction carries with it a high mortality (25%) in the first three weeks.

## CONSIDERATIONS DURING CONVALESCENT PERIOD AND AT TIME OF DISCHARGE

1. **Low-Level Exercise Testing**

   Under close supervision of trained personnel, a slow gradual increase in activity levels is started in the CCU and then continued throughout the hospital course. A low-level stress test is performed just prior to discharge in order to: 1) determine a safe level of home activity and a safe exercise prescription for outpatient cardiac rehabilitation; and 2) to identify patients at high risk for future cardiac events. Patients with a positive low-level stress test have a significant risk of cardiac - related mortality over the subsequent year(52). This subgroup should have close observation and possibly early heart catheterization and bypass surgery or PTCA.

2. **Cardiac Rehabilitation**

   One of the goals of a comprehensive rehabilitation program is to encourage risk factor modification such as cessation of smoking, dietary counseling, and treatment of hypertension and diabetes. Exercise training is also a significant component of cardiac rehabilitation and should focus on improving work capacity and reducing symptoms. The positive training effects of a lower heart rate and blood pressure reduce myocardial oxygen consumption and thus help relieve symptoms. Attention should also be given to vocational status and psychosocial manifestations of the illness. Unfortunately, cardiac rehabilitation patients have not been shown to have any significant reduction in mortality after myocardial infarction.

3. **Beta Blockers**

   The role of beta blockers in the early phase of acute myocardial infarction is unclear, although the Swedish Metoprolol Trial showed a reduction in mortality which was statistically significant at the end of the 90-day follow-up period. The majority of the reduction in mortality occurred after the first week(53).

   There are five large multicenter prospective randomized clinical trials with a total of over 11,500 patients having been tested on chronic beta blocker therapy after myocardial infarction(54). Four of these five showed significant reduction in mortality in follow-up periods varying from 3 to 24 months. Only the Sotalol Trial did not show a significant difference in treatment and placebo groups. Practolol was used in the Multicenter International Study and showed a significant reduction in mortality for those with anterior myocardial infarction. However, this drug is not used clinically because of untoward side effects.

The three remaining large trial studies are the Norwegian Multicenter Study Group (timolol, 20 mg/day), the Beta Blocker Heart Attack Trial (propranolol, 180-240 mg/day), and the Goteborg Metoprolol Trial (200 mg/day). These each showed reduced cardiac mortality regardless of the site of infarct. The decrease in mortality was primarily accounted for by significant reduction in sudden cardiac death. It is speculated that this may be due to an antiarrhythmic effect by inhibition of adrenergic stimulation.

The authors recommend that beta blockers be used in all postinfarct patients if there are no contraindications. It is suggested to begin therapy within 5 days of the myocardial infarction and to continue for at least 2 years.

The dosage schedule recommended is timolol 10 mg P.O. b.i.d., propranolol 60 to 80 mg P.O. t.i.d., or metoprolol 100 mg P.O. b.i.d. It is important to note that most patients will tolerate this treatment if the left ventricular ejection fraction is 35% or greater. Patients with borderline left ventricular function in whom congestive failure is controlled can be tried on this therapy if close follow-up can be assured.

## REFERENCES

1. DeWood MA, Spores J, Notske R, et al.: Prevalence of total coronary occlusion during the early hours of transmural myocardial infarction. N Engl J Med 303:897, 1980.

2. Oliva PB: Pathophysiology of acute myocardial infarction. Ann Intern Med 94:236, 1981.

3. Swan HJC, Shah PK: Acute myocardial infarction. In Cheng TO (ed): The International Textbook of Cardiology. New York, Pergamon Press, 1986, pp.674-709.

4. Kannel WB, Feinleib M: Natural history of angina pectoris in the Framingham study. Am J Cardiol 29:154, 1972.

5. Harvey WP: Some pertinent physical findings in the clinical evaluation of acute myocardial infarction. Circulation 40:IV-175, 1969.

6.  Dugall JC, Pryor R, Blount SG Jr: Systolic murmur following myocardial infarction. Am Heart J 87:577, 1974.

7.  Iskandrian AS, Hakki AH, Kotler MN, et al.: Evaluation of patients with acute myocardial infarction: Which test, for whom and why? Am Heart J 109:391, 1985.

8.  Goldberger AL: Myocardial Infarction: Electrocardiographic Differential Diagnosis, 3rd edition. St. Louis, C. V. Mosby, 1984.

9.  Rapaport E:  Serum enzymes and isoenzymes in the diagnosis of acute myocardial infarction. Mod Concepts Cardiovasc Dis 46:47, 1977.

10. Wagner GS:  Optimal use of serum enzyme levels in the diagnosis of acute myocardial infarction. Arch Intern Med 140:317, 1980.

11. Massie BM, Botvinick EH, Werner JA, et al.: Myocardial scintigraphy with technetium 99m stannous pyrophosphate: An insensitive test for nontransmural myocardial infarction. Am J Cardiol 43:186, 1979.

12. Taylor GJ, Humphries JO, Mellitts ED, et al.: Predictors of clinical course, coronary anatomy and left ventricular function after recovery from acute myocardial infarction. Circulation 62:960, 1980.

13. Waters DD, Forrester JS: Myocardial ischemia: Detection and quantitation. Ann Intern Med 88:239, 1978.

14. Opie LH: Myocardial infarct size. Part I. Basic considerations. Am Heart J 100:355, 1980.

15. Rude RE, Muller JE, Braunwald E: Efforts to limit the size of myocardial infarcts. Ann Intern Med 95:736, 1981.

16. McMillin-Wood JB, Bassingthwaighte JB (eds): Cardiovascular metabolic imaging: Physiologic and biochemical dynamics in vivo. Circulation 72: IV-1, 1985.

17. Schuster EH, Bulkley BH: Early post-infarction angina: Ischemia at a distance and ischemia in the infarct zone. N Engl J Med 305:1101, 1981.

18. Laffel GL, Braunwald E: Thrombolytic therapy. A new strategy for the treatment of acute myocardial infarction. N Engl J Med 311:710, 1984. A new strategy for the treatment of acute myocardial infarction. N Engl J Med 311:770, 1984.

19. Khaja F, Walton JA, Brymer JF, et al.:  Intracoronary fibrinolytic therapy in acute myocardial infarction.  Report of a randomized trial.  N Engl J Med 308:1305, 1983.

20. Rentrop KP, Feit F, Blanke H, et al.:  Effects of intracoronary streptokinase and intracoronary nitroglycerin infusion on coronary angiographic patterns and mortality in patients with acute myocardial infarction.  N Engl J Med 311:1457, 1984.

21. Stamfer MJ, Goldhaber SZ, Yusuf S, et al.:  Effect of intravenous streptokinase on acute myocardial infarction:  Pooled results from randomized trials.  N Engl J Med 307:1180, 1982.

22. TIMI Study Group:  The thrombolysis in myocardial infarction (TIMI) trial: Phase I findings.  N Engl J Med 312:932, 1984.

23. Hartzler GO, Rutherford BD, McConahay DR, et al.:  Percutaneous transluminal coronary angioplasty with and without thrombolytic therapy for treatment of acute myocardial infarction.  Am Heart J 106:965, 1983.

24. Pepine CJ, Prida X, Hill JA, et al.:  Percutaneous transluminal coronary angioplasty in acute myocardial infarction.  Am Heart J 107:820, 1984.

25. Jennings RB, Reimer KA:  Factors involved in salvaging ischemic myocardium: Effect of reperfusion of arterial blood.  Circulation 68: I-25, 1983.

26. DeSanctis RW, Block P, Hutter AM:  Tachyarrhythmias in myocardial infarction.  Circulation 45:681, 1972.

27. Chadda KD, Lichstein E, Gupta PK, et al.:  Effects of atropine in patients with bradyarrhythmia complicating myocardial infarction. Usefulness of an optimum dose for overdrive.  Am J Med 63:503, 1977.

28. Berte LE, Harrison DC:  Should prophylactic antiarrhythmic drug therapy be employed in acute myocardial infarction?  In: Rahimtoola SH (ed): Controversies in Coronary Heart Disease. Cardiovascular Clinics. Philadelphia, F. A. Davis Co., 1983, vol 13, p. 173.

29. Harrison DC:  Should lidocaine be administered routinely to all patients after acute myocardial infarction?  Circulation 58:581, 1978.

30. Norris RM, Mercer CJ:  Significance of idioventricular rhythms in acute myocardial infarction,  Progr Cardiovasc Dis 16:455, 1974.

31. Gunnar RM, Loeb HS, Scanlon PJ, et al.: Management of acute myocardial infarction and accelerating angina. Progr Cardiovasc Dis 22:1, 1979.

32. Hill NS, Antman EM, Green LH, et al.: Intravenous nitroglycerin. A review of pharmacology, indications, therapeutic effects and complications. Chest 79:69, 1981.

33. Killip T III, Kimball JT: Treatment of myocardial infarction in a coronary care unit: A two-year experience with 250 patients. Am J Cardiol 20: 457, 1967.

34. Karliner JS, Ross J Jr: Left ventricular performance after acute myocardial infarction. Progr Cardiovasc Dis 13:374, 1971.

35. Richard C, Ricome JL, Rimailho A, et al.: Combined hemodynamic effects of dopamine and dobutamine in cardiogenic shock. Circulation 67:620, 1983.

36. McCabe JC, Abel RM, Subramanian VA, et al.: Complications of intra-aortic balloon insertion and counterpulsation. Circulation 57:769,1978.

37. Cohn JN: Right ventricular infarction revisited. Am J Cardiol 43:666, 1979.

38. Klein HO, Tordjman T, Ninio R, et al.: The early recognition of right ventricular infarction: Diagnostic accuracy of the electrocardiographic V4R lead. Circulation 67:558, 1983.

39. Lopez-Sendon J, Coma-Canella I, Gamallo C: Sensitivity and specificity of hemodynamic criteria in the diagnosis of acute right ventricular infarction. Circulation 64:515, 1981.

40. Sharpe DN, Botvinick EH, Shames DM, et al.: The noninvasive diagnosis of right ventricular infarction. Circulation 57:483, 1978.

41. Dell'Italia LJ, Starling MR, Blumhardt R, et al.: Comparative effects of volume loading, dopamine, and nitroprusside with predominant right ventricular infarction. Circulation 72:1327, 1985.

42. Vlodaver Z, Edward JE: Rupture of the ventricular septum or papillary muscle complicating myocardial infarction. Circulation 55:815, 1977.

43.  Bates RJ, Beutler S, Resnekov L, et al.:  Cardiac rupture—challenge in diagnosis and management.  Am J Cardiol 40:429, 1977.

44.  Resnekov L, Chediak J, Hirsh J, et al.:  Antithrombotic agents in coronary artery disease.  Chest 89:54S, 1986.

45.  Hutchins GM, Bulkley BH:  Infarct expansion versus extension:  Two different complications of acute myocardial infarction.  Am J Cardiol 41: 1127, 1978.

46.  Baker JT, Bramlet DE, Lester RM, et al.:  Myocardial infarct extension:  Incidence and relationship to survival.  Circulation 65:918, 1982.

47.  Bulkley BH, Platia EV, Stone GA:  Ventricular aneurysm and endocardial pathology:  Relationship to malignant arrhythmias. Circulation 64:IV-306, 1981.

48.  Madigan NP, Rutherford BD, Fry RL:  The clinical course, early prognosis and coronary anatomy of subendocardial infarction.  Am J Med 60:634, 1976.

49.  Cannom DS, Levy W, Cohen LS:  The short and long-term prognosis of patients with transmural and nontransmural myocardial infarction. Am J Med 61:452, 1976.

50.  Hutter AM, DeSanctis RW, Flynn T, et al.:  Non-transmural myocardial infarction:  A comparison of hospital and late clinical course of patients with that of matched patients with transmural anterior and transmural inferior myocardial infarction.  Am J Cardiol 48:595, 1981.

51.  Marmon A, Geltman EM, Schechtman K, et al.:  Recurrent myocardial infarction:  Clinical predictors and prognostic implications. Circulation 66:415, 1982.

52.  Theroux P, Waters DD, Halphen C, et al.:  Prognostic value of exercise testing soon after myocardial infarction.  N Engl J Med 301:341, 1979.

53.  Hjalmarson A:  The Goteborg metoprolol trial in acute myocardial infarction.  Am J Cardiol 53:1D-50D, 1984.

54.  Koch-Weser J:  Beta-adrenergic blockade for survivors of acute myocardial infarction.  N Engl J Med 310:830, 1984.

# Chapter 10

# Congestive Heart Failure

Congestive heart failure (CHF) is a **symptom complex** with many different presentations and etiologies. It can be most simply defined as a pathologic condition in which impaired cardiac performance is responsible for the inability of the heart, at normal filling pressures, to increase cardiac output (CO) in proportion to the metabolic demands placed upon the circulation.

## PATHOPHYSIOLOGY

Since **CO = stroke volume (SV) x heart rate (HR)**, the variables which regulate these determinants play a role in the etiology and therapy of CHF. **Heart rate** is a reflection of the interaction between sympathetic and parasympathetic tone. **Stroke volume** is determined by three factors: preload, contractility, and afterload. These factors actually relate to isolated muscle trip performance and therefore cannot be measured accurately in the clinical setting. However, the terms are widely used in clinical practice in the following context(1):

1. **Preload.** This term refers to the passive stretch of myocardial fibers and is approximated by the ventricular end-diastolic volume. **Clinically, it is often equated with the pulmonary capillary wedge pressure (PCWP).** It is important to recognize that the **left ventricular end-diastolic pressure (LVEDP) or PCWP is inversely related to the compliance of the ventricle.** As shown in Figure 10.1, the ventricle becomes stiffer (less compliant) with ischemia or hypertrophy; therefore, a rise or fall in PCWP in a given patient may reflect changes in volume or compliance, or both.

Figure 10.1

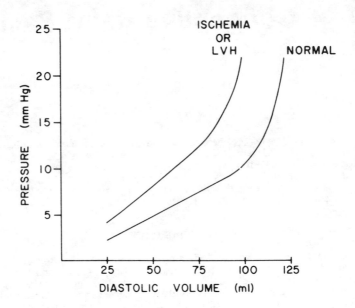

2.  **Contractility.** Refers to a reflection of the force-velocity-length relationship of the myocardium, independent of ventricular load or volume. It is often **equated with the rate of rise of ventricular pressure** (dp/dt).

3.  **Afterload.** Refers to the load or resistance encountered by the contracting myocardium, often **clinically approximated by the aortic pressure or the systemic vascular resistance.** It should be recognized that: 1) afterload is directly related to the left ventricular wall tension and is, therefore, higher in a larger ventricle, and 2) preload directly alters afterload. A stenotic aortic valve or systemic hypertension greatly increases left ventricular afterload.

When added work is imposed on the heart (i.e., hypertension, valvular disease), three principle **compensatory mechanisms** may function to help maintain CO(1):

1.  **The Frank-Starling Principle.** A myocardial muscle strip will contract with greater force if stretched to a greater resting or presystolic length. Clinical application of this principle requires substituting left ventricular end-diastolic volume (LVEDV) or LVEDP (approximated by PCWP) for fiber length and stroke work, SV, or CO for force. Frank-Starling curves relating preload (LVEDP) to force(CO)in the normal heart and in progressive left ventricular (LV) dysfunction are shown in Figure 10.2. **An impaired or failing LV requires a higher filling volume or pressure to perform the same work as does a normal ventricle.** It can be appreciated from Figure 10.2 that as the need for increased cardiac work occurs, the rise in filling presure may exceed the pulmonary capillary oncotic pressure (approximately 25 mm Hg) and pulmonary edema may ensue. Diuretics, nitrates (TNG), arterial vasodilators, and inotropic agents (digoxin, dopamine) alter the LVEDP-CO relationship and are useful in the acute and chronic management of CHF (see below).

Figure 10.2

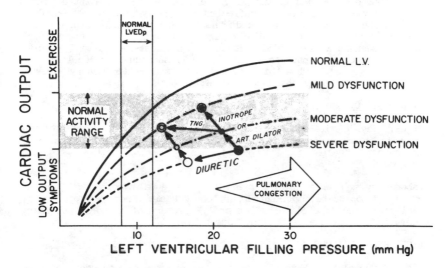

2.  **Ventricular Hypertrophy.** Hypertrophy, or an increased muscle mass, is stimulated by both pressure and volume overload states. Although hypertrophy potentially provides a beneficial increase in contractile elements, the benefits are counterbalanced by decreasing ventricular compliance which is further reduced by ischemia when the oxygen demand exceeds supply(2).

3. **Sympathetic Nervous System.** The heart is richly innervated by sympathetic fibers and the increased release of endogenous catecholamines increases contractility and heart rate(3).

## CLINICAL SIGNS AND SYMPTOMS

The major clinical manifestations of CHF can be arbitrarily divided into two categories; those due to **fluid retention** (right heart failure) and those due to **pulmonary vascular congestion** (left heart failure). This division is clinically useful but can be misleading since the right and left heart are intimately associated with each other; moreover, the most common cause of right heart failure (RHF) is left heart failure (LHF).

### LEFT HEART FAILURE

**Basic Abnormality.** Increased left atrial pressure, resulting from an elevation in LVEDP or from mitral valve disease, is transmitted to the pulmonary vascular bed and is reflected clinically by an increased PCWP. If this pressure elevation exceeds the colloid osmotic pressure of the pulmonary vascular bed, fluid accumulation within the interstitial spaces (seen as Kerley A and B lines on the chest x-ray) will result. Progression of this pathologic process will subsequently result in the accumulation of fluid within the alveolar spaces (pulmonary edema), leading to poor oxygen exchange and hypoxia.

**Symptoms.** Dyspnea, cough, orthopnea, paroxysmal nocturnal dyspnea.

**Signs.** Tachycardia and inspiratory rales (beginning at the base of the lungs and heard progressively higher as the severity of LHF increases). Expiratory wheezes due to bronchospasm (cardiac asthma) are not infrequent.

**Laboratory.** Arterial blood gas analysis may reveal hypoxemia. Chest x-ray may demonstrate prominent upper lobe vessels ("reversal of flow"), Kerley's lines, the classic "butterfly" pattern of alveolar pulmonary edema, and/or pleural effusions (see below).

### RIGHT HEART FAILURE

**Basic Abnormality.** Physiologic hormonal and renal responses occur to compensate for chronically decreased CO(4). These adaptive mechanisms lead to sodium and water retention in an effort to increase intravascular volume and  (by means of the Starling mechanism) CO.

**Symptoms.** Dyspnea on exertion, fluid retention.

**Signs.** Increased central venous pressure, hepatojugular reflux, hepatomegaly, acites, and peripheral or sacral edema may be seen.

**Laboratory.** Abnormal liver function tests may occur(5) (elevated transaminases, elevated bilirubin, prolonged prothrombin time). Pleural and pericardial effusions are not uncommon. Hyponatremia with a low urinary sodium (<20 mEq/L) ("dilutional hyponatremia") and an elevated blood urea nitrogen (BUN) are frequent and reflect a decrease in renal perfusion(4).

## RADIOLOGY OF CONGESTIVE HEART FAILURE

Irrespective of the underlying cause of CHF in an individual patient, the diagnosis of CHF must be confirmed before the initiation of any therapy. The physical examination may be very helpful, especially in RHF, but may be less helpful in diagnosing LHF since inspiratory rales may be associated with chronic lung abnormalities(6). The chest x-ray, then, becomes of clinical importance in diagnosing CHF.

### RADIOGRAPHIC STAGES OF CHF

Different radiographic stages reflecting the severity of CHF have been described(7), but the classical radiographic progression is not always seen. Moreover, the appearance and resolution rates of CHF on the chest x-ray are variable. The chest x-ray may not correlate temporally with the patient's immediate condition, i.e., there may be as much as a 12-hour diagnostic lag with the onset of CHF and a post-therapeutic lag of up to 4 days after the clinical resolution of CHF.

1. **Pulmonary Venous Congestion and Redistribution of Flow.** Normally more blood flow occurs to the dependent portions of the lungs. When the PCWP is elevated from 12 to 18 mm Hg, flow to the lower lung fields is reduced due to vasoconstriction while flow to the upper lung fields is increased. Recognition of flow distribution will be dependent upon the quality of the upright chest x-ray and is usually seen only in cases of chronic elevation of the PCW, such as in mitral stenosis.

2. **Interstitial Pulmonary Edema.** This is probably the most common radiographic sign of LHF. Fluid which accumulates in the interstitial spaces within the lung is seen as Kerley B lines (found in the lower lung fields peripherally and usually extending to the pleural surface). Fluid can also accumulate in the lobular septa which form the framework of support for the lung and is seen as Kerley A lines (found emanating from the hila outward to the lung parenchyma). The pulmonary vessels typically are somewhat enlarged and their radiographic shadows are blurred. A PCWP of 18 to 25 mm Hg is usually present.

3. **Alveolar Edema.** As the severity of the LHF increases and the PCWP rises acutely above 25 mm Hg, actual filling of the alveolar spaces with fluid can occur, i.e., pulmonary edema. This is recognized by the classic "butterfly pattern" of bilateral perihilar infiltrates.

## TWO IMPORTANT QUESTIONS WHICH MUST BE ANSWERED
## WHEN DEALING WITH CONGESTIVE HEART FAILURE

### WHAT IS THE UNDERLYING CARDIAC DISORDER?

CHF itself is **not** a diagnosis, but only a symptom complex.  Two different classifications of the etiology of CHF follow:

### Functional Classification of CHF

1.  Disorders of contractility (e.g., ischemic heart disease, cardiomyopathy).

2.  Diastolic mechanical inhibition of cardiac performance (e.g., mitral stenosis, left atrial myxoma, pericardial tamponade).

3.  Systolic mechanical ventricular overload (pressure: aortic stenosis, hypertension; volume: aortic insufficiency, mitral regurgitation).

### Anatomical Classification of CHF

1.  Valvular

2.  Systemic hypertension

3.  Pulmonary hypertension

4.  Pericardial disease

5.  Myocardial disease

6.  Congenital

7.  High-output states

8.  Traumatic (acute aortic insufficiency)

### WHAT IS THE PRECIPITATING CAUSE OF THE CHF?

Knowing the precipitating cause(s) of CHF may greatly aid in the management of the disorder.  Common precipitating factors include:

1.  Infection

2.  Pulmonary embolus

3.  Lack of medications

4.  Arrhythmias

5.  Myocardial infarction

6.  Physical stress

7.  Increased sodium intake

8.  Sodium-retaining drugs

9.  Anemia

10. Thyroid diseases

11. Bacterial endocarditis

## PULMONARY EDEMA—CLINICAL PRESENTATION

The end result of LHF may be acute pulmonary edema which is associated with considerable morbidity and mortality if not recognized quickly and treated appropriately. Since the identification of the underlying abnormality producing CHF is just as important as making the clinical diagnosis of CHF, some comments on the physical examination, ECG, and chest x-ray in regard to this end in a typical patient may be helpful.

1.  **Feel the Carotid Arteries Carefully.** The quality of the upstroke may be helpful in identifying pathologic conditions (i.e., aortic stenosis) since its rate of rise is related to left ventricular function. The carotid pulse also serves as an invaluable tool in helping to correctly identify and time any murmurs heard on auscultation of the heart.

2.  **Auscultate the Heart.** Do not let the presence of adventitious breath sounds limit your attempt to correctly identify heart sounds and murmurs. Listen for signs of **mitral stenosis** (a loud first heart sound, an opening snap best heard at the apex, and an apical diastolic rumble). Appreciation of these findings may be hindered by atrial fibrillation with a rapid ventricular response rate. A loud mid-diastolic crescendo-decrescendo murmur should alert one to the possibility of **acute aortic insufficiency**. This murmur, at times, is so loud that house staff consistently call it a systolic murmur, failing to properly time it with the carotid upstroke. A mid-systolic murmur and loud S4 gallop in the presence of sinus rhythm should alert one to the possibility of **acute mitral regurgitation**.

3.  **Examine the Electrocardiogram.** Evidence of an old or new **myocardial infarction** may be present. Atrial fibrillation in combination with large fibrillatory waves in the anterior precordial leads (V1) suggests **mitral valvular disease** with left atrial enlargement.

4. **Examine the Chest X-ray.** This is used to confirm a clinical diagnosis. Clear lung fields in the presence of a large cardiac silhouette in a dyspneic patient suggest **pericardial tamponade** (see Chapter 14).

## ACUTE PULMONARY EDEMA — THERAPY

1. Identify and eliminate any aggravating factors.

2. **High Flow Oxygen.** Best tolerated if administered by nasal prongs.

3. **Morphine Sulfate.** Use in doses of 3 to 5 mg slow IV push. This drug is beneficial in several ways:

   - Venous dilatation rapidly decreases preload.
   - Sedative effect relieves extreme anxiety.
   - Hyperventilation is decreased by directly depressing the respiratory center.

4. **Diuretics.** Rapidly acting loop diuretics (furosemide) are usually effective in doses of 40 to 80 mg IV push. Venous dilatation ensues quickly and decreases preload. An increase in urinary output will occur later(8). If no clinical response is noted after 15-30 min, double the diuretic dose and administer again.

5. **Aminophylline.** Useful if substantial bronchospasm is present (cardiac asthma). Use a loading dose of 6 mg/kg IV over 20 minutes, followed by a continuous drip of 0.2 to 0.5 mg/kg/hour. Frequently, bronchospasm will diminish with the use of oxygen, morphine sulfate, and diuretics. The use of aminophylline may precipitate arrhythmias, nausea, and vomiting.

6. **Intubation.** Indications for intubation and artificial airway control include uncontrollable and excessive secretions, marked hypoxemia, and/or severe respiratory acidosis.

7. **Sodium Bicarbonate.** Recommended only when severe metabolic acidemia is present (pH $\leq$ 7.10). The high sodium content of sodium bicarbonate may aggravate CHF.

8. **Digitalization.** Digoxin is generally not used in the acute situation. It may be useful in long-term management of CHF in patients with impaired ventricular contractility and/or volume overload(9).

9. **Dopamine and/or Dobutamine.** Potent cardiac inotropes which can be given IV and titrated to clinical response in the acute setting. Usual effective dose range is 5-15 mg/kg/min. These agents are also chronotropes and may produce arrhythmias.

## CHRONIC MANAGEMENT OF CONGESTIVE HEART FAILURE

In patients with signs and symptoms of chronic CHF, medical therapy is necessary to maximize CO yet maintain a reasonable LVEDP (15 to 20 mm Hg), thereby preventing pulmonary vascular congestion. The mainstays of medical therapy consist of:

1. **Restriction of Physical Activity.** Bedrest may sometimes be required.

2. **Low-Sodium Diet.** In patients on an extremely low sodium diet (1 gm), free water restriction may also be necessary to prevent symptomatic hyponatremia.

3. **Diuretics.** Loop diuretics (furosemide, ethacrynic acid) are most successful in doses titrated to the desired clinical effort without inducing hypotension or azotemia.

4. **Digitalization.** The increased inotropism obtained with digitalis preparations must be weighed against the side effects which can and do occur in some patients. Digoxin is the most commonly prescribed preparation. It is not metabolized by the liver but is excreted by the kidneys and has a half-life of approximately 30 hours(10). An average dose of 0.25 mg every day is used. A reduced daily dose is usually required in patients with renal failure(11). **Digitalis toxicity**(12) is more likely to occur in: 1) elderly patients, 2) renal failure, 3) small body size, 4) chronic obstructive pulmonary disease (COPD), 5) hypokalemia, or 6) digitalis in combination with quinidine(13).

The most frequent symptoms of **digitalis toxicity** are anorexia and nausea. Serum digoxin levels may be helpful in documenting toxicity but should not be overused(14), and should be drawn at least four hours after the last dose. Patients with chronic atrial fibrillation may require higher than normal "therapeutic levels" to control the ventricular rate but may not be clinically toxic. The electrocardiogram may suggest digitalis excess(12). Look for:

- Premature ventricular contractions.

- Bradycardia or atrial fibrillation with a low (<60 per min) ventricular response.

- Group beating: Implies a Wenkebach phenomenon at the level of the atrioventricular (AV) node made evident by digitalis excess.

- Regularization of the R-R interval in atrial fibrillation. Implies a junctional escape rhythm, the result of complete or intermittent AV node blockade.

5. **Vasodilator Therapy.** One often assumes that reflex compensatory mechanisms for maintaining CO and BP in the face of acute or chronic CHF will produce a favorable effect. Unfortunately, this is not always true. The increase in systemic vascular resistance (SVR) which usually occurs when CO decreases may have a deleterious effect on the heart by increasing the afterload or wall tension of the left ventricle.

**Vasodilator drugs** can frequently alter the vicious cycle of increasing SVR leading to decreased CO by decreasing total peripheral vascular resistance (TPVR) and impedance to left ventricular ejection (15). Hemodynamic improvement is the result of:

- Improved ejection fraction, which decreases LVEDP and pulmonary congestion.

- Decreased pressure work of the failing ventricle.

- Reduced wall tension, decreasing myocardial oxygen demand.

### VASODILATORS—MECHANISM OF ACTION

**Nitrates.** This class of drugs has a direct effect on the peripheral vasculature. They produce various degrees of dilatation of the systemic arterial bed (decreasing afterload) and marked dilatation of the systemic veins (decreasing preload)(11). They may also produce dilatation of the coronary arteries and possible redistribution of blood flow to the subendocardium in ischemic heart disease(16). Nitrates have no direct effect on myocardial contractility. Sublingual, oral, and intravenous preparations (40 mg of nitroglycerin dissolved in 200 cc of 5% dextrose in water [D5W]) may be used. The IV preparation has more effect on afterload than the preparations taken orally, especially at doses greater than 1.0 mcg/kg/min (see Table 10.1).

**Nitroprusside.** Administered intravenously (100 mg in 500 cc of D5W), this drug causes both arteriolar vasodilation and venodilation with resultant decrease in afterload (SVR) and a decrease in preload (PCWP)(17). Prolonged therapy (over 72 hours) can result in toxic levels of thiocyanate (>10 mg/dl) and is more likely to occur in patients with liver dysfunction.

**Hydralazine.** An effective arterial vasodilator, hydralazine is usually administered orally in combination with diuretics and/or long-acting nitrates(18). Used alone, hydralazine has little effect on preload(19). The combined regimen is generally well tolerated. Side effects include lupus-like syndrome and, occasionally, reflex tachycardia.

**Prazosin.** Prazosin is an oral vasodilating drug used for chronic preload and afterload reduction with properties similar to IV nitroprusside(20-21). Reported instances of tachyphylaxis have made its use somewhat controversial(22). However, high doses (up to 20 mg per day) and vigorous use of diuretics may alleviate this problem.

**Captopril (Capoten®).** It has been suggested that the renin-angiotensin system may be stimulated in patients with CHF and that elevated levels of angiotensin may cause an increase in systemic vascular resistance(23,24). Inhibition of angiotensin would thus be expected to reduce systemic vascular resistance, increase cardiac output, and improve overall performance. Captopril inhibits angiotensin-converting enzyme and thus attenuates the vasoconstrictor properties of the active metabolite angiotensin II. The reduction in systemic vascular resistance in CHF patients on captopril is not entirely due to the inhibition of angiotensin II. The drug also appears to inhibit degradation of bradykinin as well as decreasing sympathetic activity (reducing circulating catecholamines). Captopril is a balanced vasodilator with actions both on the arteriolar and venous beds. There is usually no increase in heart rate associated with the decrease in SVR.

Adverse effects of captopril include marked hypotension, bradycardia, skin rash, impaired renal function, and occasional cases of immune complex glomerulonephritis.

**Enalapril Maleate (Vasotec®).** This is a new angiotensin converting enzyme inhibitor which has the advantage of a once-a-day dosage schedule(25). Doses range from 2.5 mg P.O. to 5 mg P.O. once a day.

**Table 10.1**
**Afterload Reduction**

| | | | |
|---|---|---|---|
| Nitroglycerin S.L.<br>0.4-0.6 mg q2-3h | ↓ | preload | |
| Nitroglycerin P.O<br>10-40 mg q4-6h | ↓ | preload | |
| Nitroglycerin IV<br>0.2-2.0 mcg/kg/min | ↓↓ | preload & ↓ afterload | |
| Nitroprusside IV<br>0.5-10 mcg/kg/min | ↓ | preload & ↓↓ afterload | |
| Hydralazine P.O.<br>50-100 mg q6h | ↓ | afterload | |
| Prazosin P.O.<br>2-5 mg q6h | ↓ | preload & ↓ afterload | |
| Captopril P.O.<br>12.5-100 mg q12h | ↓ | preload & ↓ afterload | |
| Enalapril P.O.<br>2.5-5.0 q.d. | ↓ | preload & ↓ afterload | |

## VASODILATORS—CLINICAL USE

**Intravenous Vasodilator Agents** (nitroprusside or nitroglycerin) are indicated for use in the following situations:

1. **Acute Myocardial Infarction.** If complicated by a decrease in CO and an increase in PCWP (>18 mm Hg), IV nitroglycerin may offer an advantage over nitroprusside in this setting by producing a greater dilatory effect on myocardial collateral vessels(16,26). Vasodilator therapy may be associated with a mild decrease in BP, but diastolic pressures should not be allowed to fall below 60 mm Hg to assure adequate coronary perfusion. Reflex tachycardia usually is not a problem with commonly used doses titrated to hemodynamic response.

2. **Chronic Refractory CHF.** The use of intravenous vasodilator agents in this setting is helpful only for short-term treatment or to determine the magnitude of the hemodynamic response prior to initiating the use of long-term (P.O.) vasodilator therapy.

3. **Acute and/or Chronic Mitral Regurgitation Complicated by CHF.** IV nitroprusside in this condition can increase CO by as much as 50% and decrease PCWP without a significant change in heart rate(27).

4. **Aortic Regurgitation (Chronic or Acute) Complicated by CHF.** Nitroprusside is useful especially if hypertension is present(28).

**Oral vasodilator agents** for refractory CHF may be helpful in any patient with myocardial dysfunction (cardiomyopathy, ischemic heart disease, etc.) whose CO is decreased and PCWP is increased.

**Oral nitrates** have been shown to decrease LVEDP with only a mild concomitant decrease in BP. Cardiac output rises only slightly(29). Doses of isosorbide range from 10 mg P.O. q.i.d. to 40 mg P.O. q.i.d.

**Hydralazine,** when given orally, may produce beneficial results by increasing CO and reducing SVR and pulmonary vascular resistance. PCWP may not change dramatically, and therefore concomitant use of a diuretic or nitrates is recommended. Doses range from 25 mg P.O. b.i.d. to 100-200 mg P.O. b.i.d.

**Oral prazosin** effectively decreases preload and afterload, but tolerance to its effects must be watched for. Orthostatic hypotension may also be a problem, especially after the first dose. Starting dose is 1 mg P.O. q.d., and there is a wide range on upper limit.

**Captopril** is an angiotensin-converting enzyme inhibitor shown to be extremely effective in increasing CO and reducing SVR and may be the vasodilator of choice in chronic CHF. Doses range from 12.5 mg P.O. b.i.d. to 100 mg P.O. t.i.d.

## REFERENCES

1. Ross J Jr:  Afterload mismatch and preload reserve.  A conceptual framework for the analysis of ventricular function.  Prog Cardiovasc Dis 18:255, 1976.

2. Grossman W:  Cardiac hypertrophy:  Useful adaptation or pathologic process?  Am J Med 69:576, 1980.

3. Kent KM, Cooper T:  The denervated heart.  A model for studying autonomic control of the heart.  N Engl J Med 291:1017, 1974.

4. Cannon P:  The kidney in heart failure.  N Engl J Med 296:26, 1977.

5. Dunn GD, Hayes P, Breen KJ, et al.:  The liver in congestive heart failure.  Am J Med Sci 265:174, 1973.

6. Nath AR, Capel LH:  Inspiratory crackles—early and late.  Thorax 29:223, 1974.

7. Kostuk W, Barr JW, Simon AL, et al.:  Correlations between the chest film and hemodynamics in acute myocardial infarction.  Circulation 48:624, 1973.

8. Dikshit K, Vyden JK, Forrester JS, et al.:  Renal and extrarenal hemodynamic effects of furosemide in congestive failure after acute myocardial infarction.  N Engl J Med 288:1087, 1973.

9. Arnold SB, Byrd RC, Meister JS, et al.:  Long-term digitalis therapy improves left ventricular function in heart failure.  N Engl J Med 303:1443, 1980.

10. Doherty JE, Kane JJ:  Clinical pharmacology of digitalis glycosides.  Ann Rev Med 26:159, 1975.

11. Jelliffe RW, Brooker G:  A nomogram for digoxin therapy.  Am J Med 57:63, 1974.

12. Mason DT, Zelis R, Lee G, et al.:  Current concepts and treatment of digitalis toxicity.  Am J Cardiol 27:546, 1971.

13. Doering W:  Quinidine-digoxin interaction.  Pharmacokinetics, underlying mechanism and clinical implications.  N Engl J Med 301:400, 1979.

14. Ingelfinger JA, Goldman P:  The serum digitalis concentration—does it diagnose digitalis toxicity?  N Engl J Med 294:867, 1976.

15. Chatterjee K, Massie B, Ruben S, et al.:  Long-term outpatient vasodilator therapy of congestive failure.  Consideration of agents at rest and during exercise.  Am J Med 65:134, 1978.

16.  Chiariello M, Gold HK, Leinbach RC, et al.:  Comparison between the effects of nitroglycerin and nitroprusside on ischemic injury during acute myocardial infarction.  Circulation 54:766, 1976.

17.  Palmer RF, Lasseter KC:  Sodium nitroprusside.  N Engl J Med 292:294, 1975.

18.  Pierpont GL, Cohn JN, Franciosa JA:  Combined oral hydralazine-nitrate therapy in left ventricular failure.  Chest 73:8, 1978.

19.  Franciosa DJ, Pierpont G, Cohn JN:  Hemodynamic improvement after oral hydralazine in left ventricular failure.  Ann Intern Med 86:388, 1977.

20.  Graham RM, Pettingher WA:  Prazosin.  N Engl J Med 300:233, 1979.

21.  Mehta J, Iacona M, Feldman RL, et al.:  Comparative hemodynamic effects of intravenous nitroprusside and oral prazosin in refractory heart failure.  Am J Cardiol 41:925, 1978.

22.  Packer M, Meller J, Gorlin R, et al.:  Hemodynamic and clinical tachyphylaxis to prazosin-mediated afterload reduction in severe chronic congestive heart failure.  Circulation 59:531, 1979.

23.  Massie BM, Kramer BL, Topic N:  Lack of relationship between short-term hemodynamic effects of captopril and subsequent clinical responses.  Circulation 69:1135, 1984.

24.  Sutton FJ:  Vasodilator therapy.  Am J Med 80:54, 1986.

25.  Ayers CR:  Enalapril maleate versus captopril:  A comparison of the hormonal and antihypertensive effects.  Drugs(suppl 1):70, 1985.

26.  Armstrong PW, Walker DC, Burton JR, et al.:  Vasodilator therapy in acute myocardial infarction.  A comparison of sodium nitroprusside and nitroglycerin.  Circulation 52:1118, 1975.

27.  Goodman DJ, Rossen RM, Holloway EL, et al.:  Effects of nitroprusside on left ventricular dynamics in mitral regurgitation.  Circulation 50:1025, 1974.

28.  Bolen JL, Alderman EL:  Hemodynamic consequences of afterload reduction in patients with chronic aortic regurgitation.  Circulation 53:879, 1976.

29.  Franciosa JA, Mikulic E, Cohn JN, et al.:  Hemodynamic effects of orally administered isosorbide dinitrate in patients with congestive heart failure.  Circulation 50:1020, 1974.

# Chapter 11

# Valvular Heart Disease

## A PHYSIOLOGIC APPROACH TO BEDSIDE DIAGNOSIS

A great deal has been learned in the past two decades about cardiac pathophysiology, as a result of the proliferation of invasive (cardiac catheterization) and more recently noninvasive (echocardiography) procedures. Pressure and sound phenomena recognized at the bedside can now be correlated with cardiac catheterization data to provide logical explanations for these findings. These data have been applied in the following chapter to give the house officer the necessary basic understanding to help identify disease processes utilizing the clinical history and physical examination. A section dealing with principles of therapy has been included at the conclusion of each disease entity.

In the evaluation of an individual patient, the house officer must use the history and overall clinical setting to look for abnormal pressure waves, to perceive characteristic pressure pulses, and to listen for specific and sometimes subtle auscultatory events. By so doing, the clinical evaluation of cardiac disorders becomes extremely accurate and leads to more appropriate diagnosis and management.

In order to understand the alterations in the clinical findings imposed by valvular disease, it is useful to review briefly the **origin of normal heart sounds and pressure phenomena** (Figure 11.1). Normally, there are small gradients across the atrioventricular and semilunar valves during peak inflow and outflow, respectively. The **first heart sound** (S1) results from abrupt chordal checking of the atrial excursion of the atrioventricular (AV) valves. S1 increases in intensity when there is a rapid left ventricular (LV) pressure upstroke at the time of closure and when the P-R interval is short. A diminished rate of rise of LV pressure (LV dysfunction), a long P-R interval, or "preclosure" will diminish the intensity of the mitral first sound.

The abrupt checking of retrograde flow in the great arteries by semilunar valve closure leads to the generation of the **second sounds** (S2). The pulmonic valve closes later as the result of two phenomena: 1) later RV contraction and 2) decreased PA impedance. Increases in great vessel impedance increase the intensity of the second sound, and increases in resistance to outflow (aortic or pulmonary stenosis) will delay semilunar valve closure.

Normally, valves open silently. However, commisural fusion will result in opening sounds, termed an **opening snap** in the atrioventricular valves and an **ejection click** or ejection sound in the semilunar valves. An ejection sound can also emanate from the opening of a nonstenotic semilunar valve into a dilated root or when a markedly increased stroke volume is rapidly ejected.

A **third heart sound** (S3) or ventricular gallop will occur when there is an increase in the magnitude of early diastolic ventricular inflow, or when a normal amount of early diastolic inflow enters a poorly emptied or noncompliant ventricle. A "physiologic" S3 can be heard in persons under 25 years of age. However, an S3 usually implies disease characterized by volume overload or ventricular systolic dysfunction. An early S3 (**diastolic knock**) occurs in constrictive pericarditis.

A **fourth heart sound** (S4) or atrial gallop results from the impact of an augmented atrial contraction on a stiff or hypertrophic ventricle. Aortic or pulmonic stenosis and hypertrophic cardiomyopathy frequently manifest an S4.

The presence of both S3 and S4 implies that there is a volume overload and a need for a vigorous atrial contraction. Congestive (dilated) cardiomyopathy commonly manifests both gallop sounds. With tachycardia, S3 and S4 will fuse into a **summation gallop**.

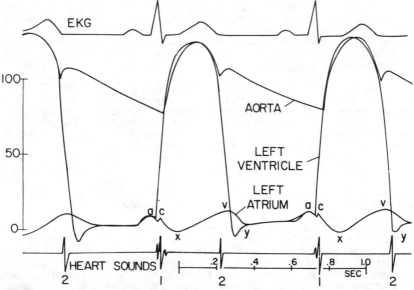

Figure 11.1  Normal Heart Sounds and Associated Pressure Phenomena

Small gradients are evident across the aortic and mitral valves only during peak left ventricular outflow and inflow. The first heart sound results from abrupt chordal checking of the atrial excursion of the atrioventricular valves at end-diastole. The abrupt cessation of retrograde flow in the great vessels by semilunar valve closure generates the second heart sound. Normally, valves open silently. The "a" wave represents atrial contraction, the "c" wave occurs at the completion of mitral valve closure, and the "v" wave results from atrial inflow while the mitral valve is closed.

## TABLE OF ABBREVIATIONS

Ao - aorta
AoV- aortic valve
AR - aortic regurgitation
AS - aortic stenosis
A2 - aortic component of the
    second heart sound
CHF- congestive heart failure
DOE- dyspnea on exertion
HR - heart rate
ICS- intercostal space
JVP- jugular venous pressure
LA - left atrium
LHF- left heart failure
LSB- left sternal border
LV - left ventricle
LVEDP-left ventricular end-
    diastolic pressure
MDM -mid-diastolic murmur
MI - myocardial infarction
MR - mitral regurgitation
MS - mitral stenosis
MV - mitral valve

NSR- normal sinus rhythm
OS - opening snap
PA - pulmonary artery
PND- paroxysmal nocturnal dyspnea
PS - pulmonary stenosis
PSM- presystolic murmur
PV - pulmonic valve
P2 - pulmonary component of the
    second heart sound
RA - right atrium
RHF- right heart failure
RSB- right sternal border
RV - right ventricle
SOB- shortness of breath
S1 - first heart sound
S2 - second heart sound
S3 - third (early diastolic) heart sound
S4 - fourth (late diastolic) heart sound
TR - tricuspid regurgitation
TS - tricuspid stenosis
TV - tricuspid valve

## MITRAL STENOSIS

### CLINICAL PRESENTATION:

DOE and/or orthopnea.
pulmonary edema with pregnancy, respiratory infection,
or atrial fibrillation.

Systemic emboli associated
with atrial fibrillation.

### PATHOPHYSIOLOGIC EXPLANATION:

The stenotic valve causes a
pressure gradient across the
mitral valve which increases
markedly at high flow rates,
raising LA pressure above pulmonary oncotic pressure. Tachycardia decreases diastolic
time and increases flow rates.

Stagnation of blood in LA leads
to thrombus formation.

Some may complain of fatigue and RHF symptoms. Usually seen in young patients with severe rheumatic involvement, often from endemic regions (Mexico, India, etc.).

"Protective" pulmonary hypertension caused by pulmonary vasoconstriction keeps cardiac output low and LA pressure does not rise. Back pressure on right heart augments TV regurgitation.

## CLINICAL/AUSCULTATORY FEATURE:

Prominent jugular "a" wave (in NSR), left parasternal lift with palpable P2.

RV is exposed to increased afterload.

Tapping/small LV impulse.

LV has decreased preload.

S1 loud and snapping (Figure 11.2).

MV closes late under high pressure with rapid LV pressure rise.

Early diastolic OS heard at base or LSB. A2-OS <80 msec indicates more severe MS.

The higher the LA pressure, the earlier the OS.

Mid-diastolic rumble heard with bell lightly applied to apical impulse. Presystolic murmur crescendos into S1.

Turbulence imparted to inflowing blood through narrow valve is accentuated as MV narrows further during presystolic closure.

Presystolic murmur may be heard in NSR and with high HRs in atrial fibrillation.

Short diastoles permit late diastolic gradient of sufficient magnitude to produce a crescendo murmur in atrial fibrillation.

Above findings may be masked or obscured in patients with pulmonary hypertension, and there may be a more prominent loud holosystolic murmur along LSB with inspiratory augmentation due to TV regurgitation.

Low flow rates may diminish intensity of S1, OS, and diastolic murmurs. TV regurgitation murmur is augmented by inspiratory increase in venous return.

A soft early diastolic blow may be heard at 2nd and  3rd left ICS (Graham Steell murmur).

Pulmonic regurgitation may result from high PA pressure and dilatation of PA.

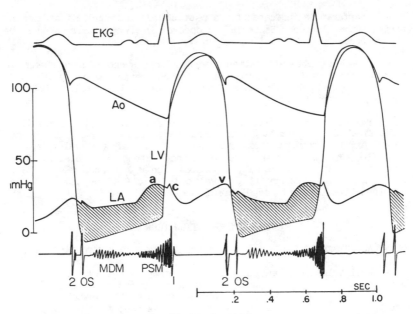

**Figure 11.2  Mitral Stenosis (Sinus Rhythm)**

There is a gradient (shaded area) between left atrial (LA) and left
ventricular (LV) pressures. The **first heart sound** (S1) is loud because the
LV pressure is high and has achieved a high rate of rise (dp/dt) at the
time of mitral valve (MV) closure.   The **opening snap** (OS) results from
abrupt deceleration of blood as it impacts against the fused commisures as
the funnel-like MV is forced open under high pressure.   The rumbling
**mid-diastolic murmur** (MDM) results from turbulence during rapid inflow.
The crescendo **presystolic murmur** (PSM) reaches maximal intensity after
the onset of atrial systole and results from closure of the MV in the face
of continued inflow which increases the velocity of flow across the
closing mitral orifice.

**THERAPY:**

   **Medical.**  If atrial fibrillation is present, control rate response
with **digoxin** and/or **propranolol** to allow for adequate diastolic filling
time.   Propranolol will be much more effective than digoxin in patients
with normal sinus rhythm to keep the heart rate from increasing with
exercise.  During periods of acute decompensation due to stress (i.e.,
pregnancy), IV propranolol is the drug of choice to control the heart

rate. **Warfarin** is indicated for a patient with a large left atrium and atrial fibrillation. Bacterial endocarditis prophylaxis should be prescribed.

Since virtually all patients with mitral stenosis have rheumatic heart disease, penicillin prophylaxis for rheumatic fever is indicated, particularly in patients exposed to high population density living or working environments.

**Surgical.** Mitral valve surgery is recommended for the Class II or III patient whose calculated mitral valve area is less than 1 $cm^2$ (normal = 4-5 $cm^2$). Commissurotomy may be possible if the valve is not calcified and subvalvular disease is not extensive. This procedure usually provides relief of mitral stenosis for at least ten years. Valve replacement is necessary if the valve is calcified or immobile, and requires life-long anticoagulation.

## MITRAL REGURGITATION (CHRONIC)

**CLINICAL PRESENTATION:**

**PATHOPHYSIOLOGIC EXPLANATION:**

Often well tolerated for many years.

LA and LV compliances adjust to volume load to produce minimal increase in LA or LV diastolic pressures. LA runoff is rapid in early diastole, decompressing pulmonary capillary pressure.

Decompensation may result from development of systemic arterial hypertension.

Slight increases in afterload will markedly increase mitral regurgitation.

**CLINICAL/AUSCULTATORY FEATURES:**

JVP often normal.

RV is not exposed to MR, since LA "v" wave builds up after RV systole is nearly complete.

Late systolic left parasternal lift. Rapid early diastolic filling wave at apex.

Expansion of LA may push the RV forward, simulating an RV lift.

S1 often obscured by a holosystolic blowing apical murmur which radiates to the axilla (Figure 11.3A).

MR begins at onset of LV systole and continues throughout systole since LV pressure exceeds that in LA throughout systole.

| Loud S3, occasionally en-compassed by short dia-stolic rumble. | Rapid early diastolic inflow from high "v" wave through non-restrictive orifice leads to rapid ventricular distention. |

## THERAPY:

**Medical.** **Digoxin** is used for its inotropic effect and, if atrial fibrillation is present, to control ventricular response. However, patients with predominant mitral regurgitation tolerate relatively fast heart rates without difficulty. Therefore, aggressive digitalization aimed at decreasing the ventricular response below 70 is seldom necessary. **Afterload reduction** (hydralazine, prazosin) is effective in decreasing the regurgitant fraction and increasing cardiac output. **Warfarin** is indicated in predominant mitral regurgitation in the setting of atrial fibrillation. Bacterial endocarditis prophylaxis is recommended. Rheumatic fever prophylaxis is indicated if the valve lesion is rheumatic.

**Surgical.** Mitral valve replacement is indicted for symptomatic patients with declining ventricular function or increasing heart size if cardiac catheterization demonstrates significant mitral regurgitation.

## MITRAL REGURGITATION (ACUTE)

| CLINICAL PRESENTATION: | PATHOPHYSIOLOGIC EXPLANATION: |
|---|---|
| May present as acute, severe respiratory distress. | Sudden volume load presented to LA and LV is poorly tolerated. |
| May follow a febrile illness, MI, or may occur spontaneously. | Ruptured chordae may complicate infective endocarditis. Rupture or infarction of papillary muscle may complicate an acute MI. |

## CLINICAL/AUSCULTATORY FEATURES:

| JVP may exhibit large "a" waves and a left parasternal lift may be present. | Right heart is exposed to mark-edly elevated right heart pressures. |
|---|---|
| Apex active, with prominent early diastolic and pre-systolic outward thrusts. S3 and S4 may both be heard, or events may be super-imposed. | Rapid early diastolic outflow from high-pressure LA, abruptly halted by noncompliant LV. |

| Apical systolic murmur begins with S1 and ends before S1 (Figure 11.3B). | Late systolic MR prevented by near equalization of LA and LV pressures. |

## THERAPY:

The accurate, early diagnosis of acute mitral regurgitation and immediate attempts at medical stabilization with afterload reduction (even if systolic pressure is normal) and diuretics are of paramount importance.   Cardiac catheterization and mitral valve replacement should quickly follow even in patients who are poor surgical candidates since the mortality of this lesion without surgery is extremely high.

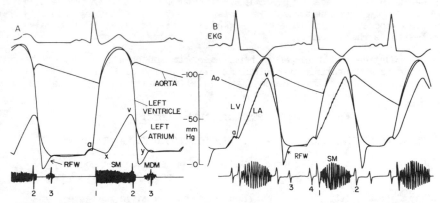

**Figure 11.3A   Chronic Mitral Regurgitation**

Mitral regurgitation produces a tall "v" wave in the left atrial (LA) pressure pulse and is accompanied by a **holosystolic murmur** (SM).   The first heart sound is attenuated.   The tall systolic "v" wave is followed by a rapid left atrial pressure drop at the onset of diastole (y descent) as blood rapidly leaves the atrium in early diastole.   A rapid filling wave (RFW) in the LV pressure trace is evident during early diastole and is accompanied by a third heart sound(S3).   A mid-diastolic murmur (MDM) may be heard during rapid early diastolic inflow from the high-pressure LA and may simulate the murmur of rheumatic mitral stenosis.

**Figure 11.3B   Acute Mitral Regurgitation**

"Ventricularization" of the atrial pressure pulse (giant "v" wave) is caused by acute regurgitation into a noncompliant left atrium and is usually the result of acute chordal or papillary muscle rupture. There is a rapid filling wave (RFW) in the LV pressure contour associated with a third heart sound (S3). A fourth heart sound (S4) accompanies atrial contraction ("a" wave). A systolic murmur (SM) can be heard and stops before the second sound (S2) because the LA pressure has nearly achieved the same level as the LV pressure.

## MITRAL VALVE PROLAPSE

**CLINICAL PRESENTATION:**

**PATHOPHYSIOLOGIC EXPLANATION:**

Thin, anxious young female with palpitations, chest pain, fatigue, syncope. Less frequently symptomatic in males.

Atrial and ventricular tachyarrhythmias common. Myocardium may be ischemic due to abnormal tension on papillary muscle. Autonomic dysfunction may cause syncope.

May present as transient ischemic attacks or stroke.

Emboli may occur from platelet aggregations on leaflets (rare).

May present as acute MI.

Mechanism unknown. Coronary emboli or spasm postulated.

May present with acute cardiac decompensation.

Ruptured chordae due to poor connective tissue integrity.

Less Common Symptoms:

- Sudden death

- Ventricular fibrillation

- Progressive dyspnea

- Progressive regurgitation

- Fever, malaise after dental procedure

- Bacterial endocarditis

Often tall, thin, with high-arched palate. Pectus excavatum, straight back, or kyphoscoliosis. Joints often hyperextensible.

Some cases may represent a systemic connective tissue disorder. (Marfan's disease, Ehlers-Danlos, etc.)

Dynamic apex with mid-systolic retraction. Variably timed mid-systolic click followed by late systolic murmur (Figure 11.4), earlier with standing, later with squatting.

The mitral valve is "too big" for the left ventricle, and after initial competent coaptation (Figure 11.5), inflation and slippage of the redundant leaflets (prolapse) are halted by chordal restraints.

The abrupt cessation of slippage causes audible click and palpable mid-systolic apical retraction, followed by mitral regurgitation (usually trivial) which causes the murmur. Perturbations which decrease the size of the LV (e.g., standing) exaggerate the ventriculo-valvular disproportion and lead to an earlier click and murmur. Squatting increases LV size and prolapse occurs later in systole.

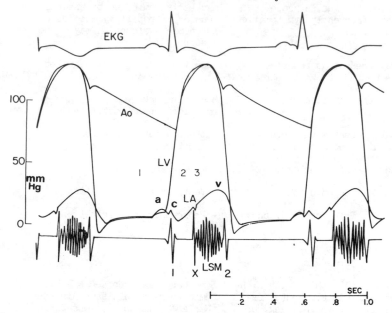

**Figure 11.4  Mitral Valve Prolapse (Hemodynamics)**

Aortic (Ao), left ventricular (LV), and left atrial (LA) pressures are usually normal with insignificant mitral regurgitation. The onset of prolapse and regurgitation are dependent on achieving a critical LV volume. Postural changes (squatting, passive leg raising) and pharmacologic interventions (phenylephrine), which increase preload and afterload, respectively, cause the click (X) and systolic murmur to occur later in systole. Standing after squatting (decreased preload), a

Valsalva maneuver (decreased preload), and amyl nitrate (decreased afterload) result in an early systolic click followed by an accentuated murmur.

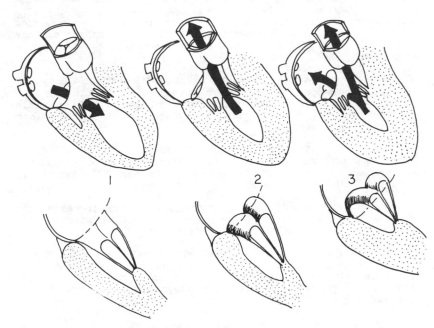

**Figure 11.5 Mitral Valve Prolapse (Anatomy)**

Mitral valve prolapse occurs when the distance between the basal and papillary muscle attachments of the elongated leaflet(s) become sufficiently short to permit the leaflet(s) to "overinflate" during systole and move toward the left atrium. The first drawings (1) in this figure demonstrate the LV contour and mitral leaflet position during diastole. The middle figure (2) depicts the LV silhouette and mitral leaflet position in early systole; the papillary muscle has shortened and maintains the leaflet at the position of the mitral annulus. As systole continues (3), a redundant leaflet will "overinflate" once the distance between the annulus and papillary muscles reaches a critical dimension. Prolapse then ensues, causing the valve to be incompetent in mid-to-late systole.

## THERAPY:

Propranolol, in doses from 40 to 320 mg/day, has been effective in controlling the "adrenergic" symptoms such as tachycardia, palpitations, and anxiety-provoked arrhythmias. It is thought that some of the arrhythmias may have their basis in the abnormal stresses put on the valve leaflets and papillary muscles by the prolapsing valve. By decreasing the ventriculo-valvular disproportion, the amount of mitral prolapse may be reduced. This effect may explain the drug's utility in lessening arrhythmias.

Some arrhythmias may require additional antiarrhythmic agents such as diphenylhydantoin (for ventricular extrasystoles) or quinidine (for atrial fibrillation). Because of the tendency towards long QT intervals in mitral prolapse, quinidine should not be used as a first-line drug to treat ventricular ectopy.

Chest pain and fatigue are more difficult symptoms to control. Often, reassuring the patient (when appropriate) that she or he does not have coronary artery disease, combined with treatment with propranolol, can improve otherwise incapacitating symptoms.

We believe that antibiotic prophylaxis for dental procedures and potentially "dirty" surgery is indicated in all patients with auscultatory evidence of mitral prolapse.

Some surgeons have claimed that mitral valve plication and/or annuloplasty may improve disabling symptoms even in patients with hemodynamically insignificant mitral valve regurgitation. These observations suggest that the valve plays a primary role in the symptomatology.

## AORTIC REGURGITATION (CHRONIC)

| CLINICAL PRESENTATION: | PATHOPHYSIOLOGIC EXPLANATION: |
| --- | --- |
| Often well tolerated for years despite evidence of significant cardiac enlargement. | LV dilates to accept volume load without increasing filling pressure. |
| Angina may be major limitation. | Low coronary perfusion pressure and increased LV wall tension may cause supply/demand imbalance. |
| Orthopnea or PND more common than DOE | Prolonged diastoles (slow HR) overfill the ventricle, and accentuate supply/demand imbalance. |

## CLINICAL/AUSCULTATORY FEATURES:

Bounding pulses (head bobbing, capillary pulse, etc.). Systolic hypertension, low (<50) diastolic pressure. Displaced apical impulse with rapid filling wave.

Rapid runoff lowers diastolic pressure, increases stroke volume, pulse pressure, and systolic pressure. LV fills rapidly from mitral inflow and Ao backflow.

Loud ejection click at apex, transmitted to base (Figure 11.6A).

Vigorous opening of aortic valve to initiate ejection of increased stroke volume.

S3 at apex.

Increased early diastolic filling of LV.

### Four Murmurs May Be Heard:

- Early peaking, harsh, mid-systolic "ejection" murmur at the base.

Increased systolic stroke volume rapidly ejected produces flow murmur in LV outflow tract.

- Decrescendo diastolic blow along sternum to apex. If aortic root markedly dilated, murmur may be louder along right sternal border.

Ao backflow toward LV diminishes in late diastole. Aneurysmal dilatation of Ao often produces murmur on the right.

- Apical mid-diastolic rumble and pre-systolic accentuation (Austin Flint murmur).

Aortic regurgitation impinges on anterior mitral leaflet and decreases effective orifice size in mid-diastole. Atrial contraction "kicks" mitral valve open to compete with aortic regurgitation for filling of ventricle in presystole.

- Apical early systolic "purified" ejection murmur.

"Filtering effect" of myocardium smoothes out low frequency components of ejection murmur.

## THERAPY:

**Medical.** Digitalis and subacute bacterial endocarditis (SBE) prophylaxis are indicated. Afterload reduction is indicated if hypertension is present. Noninvasive evaluation may be done at regular intervals to assess the severity of the aortic regurgitation and the left ventricular function. Clues to the increasing severity of the AR and decline in LV function include: a history of paroxysmal nocturnal dyspnea, the presence of increasing pulse pressure (>100 mm Hg) or diminishing aortic diastolic pressure (<50 mm Hg), a loud, solitary mid-diastolic Austin Flint murmur, an S3, increasing cardiomegaly, increasing internal LV dimensions (systolic internal diameter of >5.5 cm on echocardiogram), and a declining ejection fraction at rest or with exercise.

**Surgical.** Optimal timing of aortic valve replacement is important to prevent irreversible myocardial damage. If consideration of the above parameters indicates severe AR and/or LV dysfunction, confirmed at cardiac catheterization, aortic valve replacement is recommended. Post-operative studies have shown a decrease in heart size with improved LV function.

## AORTIC REGURGITATION (ACUTE)

**CLINICAL PRESENTATION:**

**PATHOPHYSIOLOGIC EXPLANATION:**

Frequently seen in IV drug addicts associated with fever and embolic episodes. Severe dyspnea, tachypnea, and orthopnea.

Infective endocarditis (especially Staphylococcus aureus) rapidly destroys leaflet tissue and LV is suddenly presented with an intolerable volume load.

**CLINICAL/AUSCULTATORY FEATURES:**

Pulses may not be bounding, diastolic pressure may be >50 with normal pulse pressure.

Stroke volume not markedly increased. Elevated LVEDP "buoys up" aortic diastolic pressure.

S1 soft or absent. Loud mid-diastolic murmur may obscure soft diastolic blow (Figure 11.6B).

MV precloses in mid-diastole (may be confirmed by echocardiogram).

Aortic regurgitant murmur may be of short duration.

Early equilibration of LV and aortic pressures terminates regurgitant flow in mid-diastole.

**THERAPY:**

Acute aortic regurgitation is a potentially reversible illness which carries a poor prognosis if treated by medical means alone. Prompt clinical diagnosis (physical exam and echocardiograms are most helpful), medical stabilization (bedrest, diuretics, afterload reduction), and early surgical intervention usually lead to a favorable outcome. Even in the setting of active bacterial endocarditis, aortic valve replacement must not be postponed if decompensation is present.

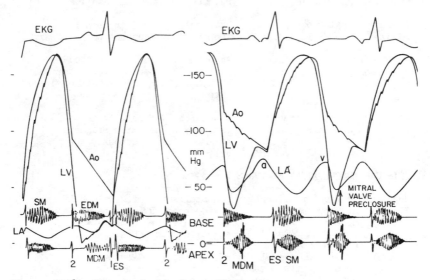

**Figure 11.6A Chronic Aortic Regurgitation**

A low aortic diastolic pressure, a wide pulse pressure, and a rapid aortic upstroke are characteristic findings. On auscultation, a harsh early peaking systolic murmur (SM) and decrescendo early diastolic murmur (EDM) are heard at the 2nd right intercostal space and along the left sternal border. At the cardiac apex, a mid-to-late-diastolic murmur (MDM) (Austin Flint murmur) may be heard as well as an ejection sound or click (ES). The presence of third and fourth heart sound will be determined by the state of left ventricular compliance.

**Figure 11.6B Acute Aortic Regurgitation**

Aortic diastolic pressure and pulse pressure are usually normal. The LV end-diastolic pressure is characteristically elevated and serves to "buoy up" aortic diastolic pressure. An early peaking systolic murmur (SM) may be heard at the base and apex. The early equilibration of LV and aortic pressures during diastole results in a soft decrescendo diastolic murmur of short duration. When regurgitation is severe, LV pressure exceeds left atrial (LA) pressure during diastole, resulting in early closure or preclosure of the mitral valve. Preclosure is accompanied by a mid-diastolic murmur (MDM), heard best at the apex, which is thought to result from mitral valve closure during high velocity left atrial inflow. With preclosure, the first heart sound is soft or absent.

## AORTIC STENOSIS

| CLINICAL PRESENTATION: | PATHOPHYSIOLOGIC EXPLANATION: |
|---|---|
| Postexertional chest pain or syncope.  CHF late sign. | Myocardial $O_2$ consumption is increased by pressure work. |
| Atrial fibrillation tolerated poorly. | Arrhythmias poorly tolerated because LV hypertrophied, atrial kick important to maintain cardiac output. |
| May not cause symptoms until 7th or 8th decade. | Acquisition of calcium in leaflets may worsen mild stenosis or immobilize previously normal valve. |

### CLINICAL AUSCULTATORY FEATURES:

| | |
|---|---|
| Jugular "a" waves prominent. Slow-rising, low-amplitude carotid pulse pressure. | Noncompliant, thick-walled LV may decrease RV compliance. Stenotic valve "damps" LV ejection into aorta. |
| Powerful, sustained apical systolic impulse, with pre-systolic outward thrust and prominent S4. | LV contraction "isometric" throughout systole.  Concentric hypertrophy renders LV noncompliant and increases strength of "a" wave kick. |
| S2 may split paradoxically. | Systole prolonged by obstruction. |
| Loud early systolic ejection sound (click) at apex (Figure 11.7A) which diminishes with age ( Figure 11.7B). | If valve mobile, check of upward doming causes click. Click disappears if valve immobilized by calcium. |
| Late-peaking crescendo-decrescendo harsh murmur at 2nd right ICS transmitted to carotids, modified (smoother) murmur at apex. | Maximum murmur intensity occurs at time of maximum LV/Ao pressure gradient, later with severe stenosis.  Apical transmission "filtered" by myocardium. |

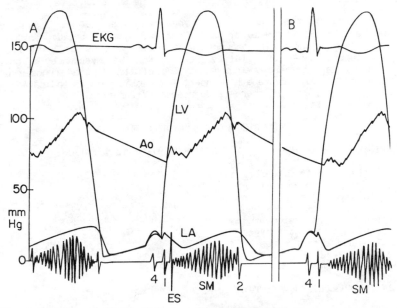

**Figures 11.7A and 11.7B   Valvular Aortic Stenosis**

A pressure gradient between the left ventricle (LV) and aorta (Ao) is characteristically present and associated with a crescendo-decrescendo systolic murmur (SM).   If the aortic cusps are mobile, an ejection sound or click (ES) may precede the systolic murmur.   With decreasing cusp mobility, ES decreases in intensity (11.7B).   The intensity of the murmur will depend upon valve area, the recorded gradient, cardiac output, and blood viscosity.   LV hypertrophy and altered LV compliance result in third and fourth heart sounds.

**THERAPY:**

A most useful diagnostic test in the elderly (>60-year-old) patient with suspected aortic stenosis is cardiac fluoroscopy.   Significant aortic stenosis will almost invariably demonstrate a **calcified** and **immobile** aortic valve.   Since mitral annular calcification may simulate the murmur of aortic stenosis, this condition can be ruled in or out.   If the coronary arteries are heavily calcified and there is little or no valve calcification, coronary artery disease with papillary muscle dysfunction simulating the murmur of aortic stenosis should be suspected. Echocardiography and Doppler will help confirm the diagnosis.

Critical aortic stenosis (AoV area less than 1.0 $cm^2$) usually presents with one or more of the classical symptom triad: angina, syncope, and dyspnea. The occurrence of these symptoms implies a poor prognosis with a 5-year mortality greater than 50%, even under optimal medical therapy. Therefore, confirmation of the aortic stenosis by cardiac catheterization and subsequent AoV replacement is indicated in these patients, even if there is decreased LV function.

## TRICUSPID VALVE DISEASE

**CLINICAL PRESENTATION:**          **PATHOPHYSIOLOGIC EXPLANATION:**

Typically patients with rheumatic TS or TR have concomitant MV disease, and their symptoms are caused predominantly by their left heart lesions and/ or resulting pulmonary hypertension. Important clues to the presence of tricuspid disease are outlined.

### CLINICAL/AUSCULTATORY FEATURES:

Prominent Jugular Venous Pulsations:

- Large "a" waves and a diminished"y"descent (Figure 11.8).

  Diastolic and pre-systolic gradient across tricuspid valve.

- Large "v" waves with rapid y descent in TR. Liver enlarged and pulsatile.

  Systolic regurgitation increases RA volume, early diastolic run-off unimpeded.

- Not infrequently, "v" waves are not prominent despite massive regurgitation.

  RA and systemic venous capacitance may increase sufficiently to "absorb" large volume of regurgitation without large pressure swings.

Inspiratory increase in
murmur intensity.

Negative intrathoracic pressure
augments systemic venous return.

- Diastolic and pre-
  systolic murmur in
  TS (Figure 11.8).

- Holosystolic murmur
  in TR.

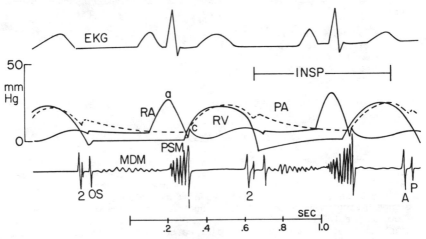

**Figure 11.8 Tricuspid Stenosis**

Prominent jugular venous "a" waves, an opening snap (OS), and a presystolic murmur (PSM) along the left sternal border which increases with
inspiration (insp) are characteristic auscultatory findings. Right
heart catheterization will reveal a diastolic gradient between the RA and
RV and an attenuated "y" descent.

**THERAPY:**

The impact of tricuspid regurgitation is greater when there is
pulmonary hypertension, often present due to concomitant mitral valve
disease. If the mitral valve must be replaced and there is organic
tricuspid regurgitation, the residual stenosis inherent in the
prosthetic valve maintains a high pulmonary arterial pressure,
especially with exercise. Therefore, tricuspid valve annuloplasty or

replacement is often required in combined mitral and tricuspid disease. Severely symptomatic tricuspid stenosis usually requires valve replacement since commissurotomy is rarely successful. Concomitant mitral stenosis is almost invariably present, but its signs and symptoms may be masked by the low output through the right heart.

## SIMULATORS OF VALVULAR HEART DISEASE

A careful history and bedside examination of the patient with presumed valvular heart disease (VHD) usually leads the physician to a preliminary diagnosis. However, one must keep in mind certain other disease entities which tend to simulate classical valvular heart disease. These include:

- Aortic sclerosis.
- Left atrial myxoma.
- Constrictive pericarditis.
- Congestive cardiomyopathy.
- Hypertrophic cardiomyopathy.

A summary of these entities and how they may be differentiated from VHD follows.

## AORTIC SCLEROSIS

Elderly patients are frequently found to have systolic ejection murmurs at the base of the heart, and may have aortic valvular calcification visible by fluoroscopy. Since it is not uncommon for elderly patients to have one or more of the classic triad of aortic stenosis symptoms (angina, syncope, and failure), the clinician may be faced with a difficult clinical decision--whether or not the patient has significant **aortic stenosis.** Cardiac catheterization carries a higher risk of complications in the elderly, and it is to be avoided if aortic stenosis can be ruled out by noninvasive means.

**Clinical Examination.** A full volume and normal upstroke of the carotid pulse  plus an intact aortic closure sound mitigate against significant aortic stenosis in an elderly patient. However, a rigid arterial system may transmit a brisk upstroke to the carotid pulse and thus obscure a valuable sign of significant aortic stenosis. On the other hand, a failing myocardium in degenerative heart disease may produce a 4th heart sound and slow carotid upstroke which simulate aortic stenosis.

Cardiac fluoroscopy may be useful in differentiating aortic stenosis (in which the heavily calcified leaflets fail to open wide in systole) from aortic sclerosis (in which a wide systolic opening of mildly calcified leaflets may be demonstrated). Echocardiography is often disappointing since the aortic valve region is echo-dense in both aortic sclerosis and stenosis.

## LEFT ATRIAL MYXOMA

### CLINICAL PRESENTATION:

Intermittent pulmonary
congestion ("pneumonia"),
embolic episodes. Posi-
tional symptoms. Elevated
sedimentation rate, fever.

### PATHOPHYSIOLOGIC EXPLANATION:

Positional ball-valve effect
if tumor pendunculated.
Tumor friable and fragments
easily.

### CLINICAL/AUSCULTATORY FEATURES:

Elevated JVP, RV lift.
Loud P2. Early systolic
apical retraction; late
loud S1. Early diastolic
thudding sound ("tumor
plop")(Figure 11.9).
Variable systolic and
diastolic murmurs.

Pulmonary hypertension (caused
by increased LA pressure) common. Tumor movement from LV to
LA and LA to LV produce loud
sounds. "Wrecking ball" effect
of tumor on MV may produce MR.
Ball-valve effect causes MS.

**Echocardiography** should be done whenever myxoma is suspected. It is
usually diagnostic.

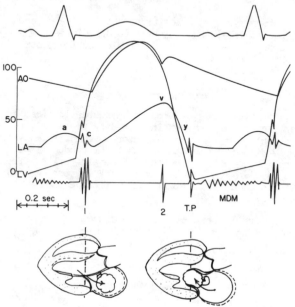

**Figure 11.9  Left Atrial Myxoma**

Left heart catheterization may reveal a large pressure gradient between the LA and LV and tall "a" and "v" waves suggestive of mitral stenosis and regurgitation. However, the downslope of the "v" wave, or "y" descent, is very rapid and followed by an early diastolic "notch" and attenuated LA pressure drop. The pressure notch may be synchronous with an early diastolic sound or "tumor plop" (TP) caused by the movement of a pedunculated, mobile myxoma into the mitral valve orifice. In this position, the tumor mass impedes left atrial outflow.

## CONSTRICTIVE PERICARDITIS

**CLINICAL PRESENTATION:**

Marked right-sided failure, usually with ascites and tender hepatomegaly. Atrial

**PATHOPHYSIOLOGIC EXPLANATION:**

Pericardial constriction causes equal elevation of diastolic filling pressure in all four

fibrillation is common. Heart size may be normal or minimally enlarged. Pericardial calcification best seen on lateral x-ray.

chambers. Manifestations of right heart failure occur at lower filling pressure on right side because of added hydrostatic pressure on compartments below the thorax.

## CLINICAL/AUSCULTATORY FEATURES:

Markedly elevated JVP with rapid early diastolic dip and plateau. Apical impulse may exhibit exaggerated early diastolic outward thrust and systolic retraction. Early diastolic sound ("knock") may be loudest heart sound. (See Chapter 14, Figure 14.2.)

Early diastolic inflow into restricted ventricles from high pressure atria is rapid initially, but then abruptly cut off by inability of ventricles to expand. The pressure events (Figure 14.2) reveal an early diastolic dip and late diastolic plateau representing these two phases, and the pericardial knock marks the transition between rapid and restricted inflow.

## THERAPY:

Since constrictive pericarditis may emulate advanced liver disease, nephrotic syndrome, and protein-losing enteropathy, a strong clinical suspicion (and observation of the neck veins) should lead the clinician to the appropriate evaluation by cardiac catheterization. Pericardectomy is the appropriate treatment and provides marked symptomatic improvement.

## CONGESTIVE (DILATED) CARDIOMYOPATHY

### CLINICAL PRESENTATION:

### PATHOPHYSIOLOGIC EXPLANATION:

Dyspnea, chest pain, peripheral edema. Evidence of systemic and/or pulmonary emboli. Recent past history of excessive alcohol ingestion, viral illness, development of symptoms in peripartum period.

Dilated, poorly contractile ventricles have high filling pressure and increased work. Stagnant flow promotes mural thrombi. Alcohol or pregnancy may predispose to cardiac damage from toxins or unknown factors when host resistance is lowered.

### CLINICAL/AUSCULTATORY FEATURES:

Elevated JVP, diffuse precordial pulsations over both ventricles with rapid

Biventricular failure. Low ejection fraction causes increased end-systolic volume and reduces filling wave, and/or pre-systolic wave. Poor quality S1, loud gallop(s), variable holosystolic murmur over apex or LSB.

compliance to atrial inflow. Poor contractility reduces mitral closing velocity. Functional AV valve incompetence due to dilated ventricles and papillary muscle dysfunction.

**Echocardiography** can be diagnostic when enlarged and poorly contractile ventricles are demonstrated.

**THERAPY:**

Optimum medical management, including bedrest, diuretics, and afterload agents, is necessary. Surgical treatment is limited to heart transplant, currently being performed on a limited basis in young patients without pulmonary hypertension or other organ damage after careful patient selection.

## HYPERTROPHIC CARDIOMYOPATHY (HCM)

**CLINICAL PRESENTATION:**

**PATHOPHYSIOLOGIC EXPLANATION:**

History of unexpected sudden death in family. Dyspnea, chest pain, syncope. Poor tolerance to tachycardia, exercise, or atrial fibrillation.

Many cases are familial with dominant autosomal inheritance. Thick, poorly compliant LV has high energy requirements, requires long diastoles to fill adequately and to sustain output.

**CLINICAL/AUSCULTATORY FEATURES:**

Elevated "a" waves in JVP. Jerky carotid pulses. Sustained late systolic LV impulse preceded by presystolic thrust. Loud S4, variable mid-late systolic murmur at apex and LSB, poorly transmitted to carotids. Murmur increases with standing and Valsalva manuever. (See Chapter 13, Figure 13.1).

Decreased biventricular diastolic compliance with rapid systolic ejection. Ventricle empties rapidly and completely (ejection fraction often 90%) with late systolic isometric contraction. Murmur may be due to late systolic narrowing of outflow tract and/or MR as contracted ventricle distorts MV, made worse by pathologically small LV volume.

**THERAPY:**

Propranolol, in doses above 320 mg/day, is usually effective in controlling symptoms. Calcium-blocking agents (verapamil, nifedipine) have been used on a limited number of patients with encouraging results.

Surgical treatment (septal myotomy) has been advocated when severe symptoms are intractable to medical therapy. The relatively high surgical and postoperative mortality (10-15%) and the failure of this therapy to improve the mortality statistics over medical therapy render surgical therapy less effective in HCM than in valvular disease.

## SUGGESTED READINGS

1.  Chizner MA, Pearle DL, de Leon AC:  The natural history of aortic stenosis in adults, Am Heart J 99:419-424, 1980.

2.  Criley JM, Chambers RD, Blaufuss AH, et al.:  Mitral stenosis: Mechanico-acoustical events.  In:  The Physiologic Principles of Heart Sounds and Murmurs. American Heart Association Monograph. 1974.  Dallas, Texas.

3.  Criley JM, Heger J:  Prolapsed mitral leaflet syndrome.  In: Congenital Heart Disease in Adults. Cardiovascular Clinics. Philadelphia, F.A. Davis Co., pp. 213-233.

4.  Fontana ME, Kissel GL, Criley JM:  Functional anatomy of mitral valve prolapse.  In:  The Physiologic Principles of Heart Sounds and Murmurs.   American Heart Association Monograph. October 1975. Dallas, Texas.

5.  Goldschlager N, Pfeifer J, Cohn K, et al.:  The natural history of aortic regurgitation:  A clinical and hemodynamic study, Am J Med 54:577-588, 1973.

6.  Johnson AD, Engler RL, LeWinter M, et al.:  The medical and surgical management of patients with aortic valve disease--a symposium. West J Med 126:460-478, 1977.

7.  Moganroth J, Perloff JK, Zeldis SM, et al.:  Acute severe aortic regurgitation:  Pathophysiology, clinical recognition, and management, Ann Intern Med 87:223-232, 1977.

8.  Roberts WC, Perloff JK:  Mitral valvular disease:  A clinico-pathologic survey of the conditions causing the mitral valve to function abnormally, Ann Intern Med 77:939-975, 1972.

9.  Roberts WC, Perloff JK, Constantino T:  Severe valvular aortic stenosis in patients over 65 years of age:  A clinicopathologic study, Am J Cardiol 27:497-506, 1977.

10. Ronan JA, Steelman RB, de Leon AC, et al.:  The clinical diagnosis of acute severe mitral insufficiency, Am J Cardiol 27:284-290, 1971.

# Chapter 12

# Congenital Heart Disease

## INTRODUCTION--AN OVERVIEW

Since many patients who survive to adulthood with congenital heart disease are potentially operable, and the natural history of many congenital heart disease lesions, particularly those with either high pulmonary blood flow or with cyanosis, is associated with progressive disability and premature death, it is important for the house officer to recognize the need to establish a presumptive diagnosis and initiate steps leading to a definitive diagnosis. Patients with cyanotic congenital heart disease disorders are especially under a Sword of Damocles; the potential for hyperuricemia, increased blood viscosity, paradoxical embolism, and cerebral infarction or abscess is all too often realized(1-8).

Congenital heart disease (CHD) may permit survival into adult life because of certain favorable factors:

1. The lesion is mild.
2. Multiple lesions counterbalance one another.
3. Compensatory mechanisms have taken place. .
4. The lesions have been surgically corrected or palliated.

At the same time, certain complications may take place which render the clinical presentation less clear in the adult with CHD than in the child:

1. Acquired valvular, vascular, or myocardial disease.
2. Infective endocarditis.
3. Embolic phenomena.
4. Pulmonary hypertension.
5. Congestive failure.
6. Arrhythmias.
7. Surgical misadventures.

A well-focused noninvasive workup with the availability of the imaging capability of contemporary echographic, Doppler, scintigraphic, and magnetic resonance imaging technology is capable of establishing a definitive diagnosis in the majority of cases.  In many instances, the anatomical information established by noninvasive means is sufficiently accurate to render invasive procedures redundant.  It is important to emphasize the necessity for a presumptive diagnosis not only in choosing the appropriate diagnostic modalities but in guiding their application. An unfocused diagnostic effort may yield ambiguous or misleading results.

The diagnostic value of the history, cardiac physical examination, and the "routine" laboratory tests will be emphasized in this chapter. The choice of appropriate secondary (specialized noninvasive) and tertiary (invasive) studies should take into consideration the differential diagnostic possibilities afforded by the clinical evaluation.

The secondary diagnostic studies permit detection and quantitation, and to a lesser extent, localization of shunts.  For example, radionuclide scintigraphy can rule in right-to-left shunts by detection of intravenously injected radiolabeled microspheres in the renal parenchyma, but cannot localize the site of shunting.  Similarly, intravenous injection of a radionuclide that can be tracked by placement of scintigraphic cursors over the lung fields will detect early recirculation curves compatible with left-to-right shunting, but cannot distinguish the site of shunting.  These radionuclide studies may falsely diagnose shunts when there is delayed transit through the right heart due to tricuspid regurgitation or when certain high flow states are present.

Two-dimensional (2D) echocardiography can define atrial and ventricular septal defects but can be falsely positive in suggesting atrial defects because of echo "dropout" and can miss ventricular septal defects and right ventricular outflow obstruction.

"Color flow doppler imaging," a technique in which 2D echocardiography   is combined with color-coded signals which designate flow toward and flow away from the transducer, as well as high velocity or turbulent flow, may almost eliminate the need for angiography in critically ill infants and some adults.  Once again, a strong presumption of congenital heart disease and a specific differential diagnosis should be present to utilize this technique appropriately.

Magnetic resonance imaging (MRI) can render superb images of the heart, particularly when the image acquisition is gated to the electrocardiogram and appropriate image planes ("slices") are utilized.

It is the purpose of this chapter to alert the physician to the more common forms of CHD which may be encountered in the adult (2,6,7). Because surgical techniques have evolved, rendering more and more patients with CHD amenable to palliative or corrective surgery(3), a high index of suspicion of CHD is warranted when patients' cardiac findings cannot be explained on the basis of acquired heart disease.

## RECOGNITION OF CONGENITAL HEART DISEASE

A significant CHD lesion will usually present with two or more of the following findings:

1. A precordial murmur.  (If the murmur is continuous, a diagnosis of CHD is virtually assured.)
2. Chamber enlargement or hypertrophy.
3. Abnormal pulmonary vascularity on chest roentgenogram.
4. Abnormal cardiac silhouette on chest roentgenogram.
5. Cyanosis with or without clubbing or polycythemia.
6. Abnormal ECG.

## CLASSIFICATION OF CONGENITAL HEART DISEASE

### ANATOMICAL ABNORMALITIES

There are three basic **anatomical** or **structural** abnormalities which may be present singly or in combination in an adult patient with CHD:

1. **Obstruction** to transvalvar or great artery flow.  (If **obstruction** is complete, it is termed **atresia**.)
2. **Communication** between chambers or great vessels.
3. **Transposition** of great arteries and/or veins.  (This category also includes anomalous connection of systemic veins to the left heart or pulmonary veins to the right heart.)

### FUNCTIONAL ABNORMALITIES

These anatomical abnormalities in turn lead to four types of **functional** abnormalities which may also occur alone or in combination:

1. Ventricular or atrial enlargement or hypertrophy.
2. Systemic or pulmonary hypertension.
3. Left to right shunting:  Pulmonary blood flow (PBF) > systemic blood flow (SBF).
4. Right to left shunting:  Arterial $O_2$ desaturation with SBF > PBF.

## PATHOPHYSIOLOGY

Since it is the functional sequelae that usually permit clinical recognition of CHD, it is important to understand the inter-relationships between the anatomical defects and the functional results.

1. **OBSTRUCTIONS** to ventricular outflow or great vessel flow produce a pressure drop (gradient) across the obstruction with a higher-than-normal pressure and hypertrophy of the upstream ventricle.  Obstruction to ventricular inflow leads to dilatation and hypertrophy of the upstream atrium.

A.   The pressure gradient across a stenotic outflow tract is associated with increased velocity (gradient = 4 x velocity$^2$), and murmur intensity is proportional to velocity to the fourth power.   Therefore, a long, late peaking murmur suggests severe stenosis since it implies a long, late-peaking gradient.

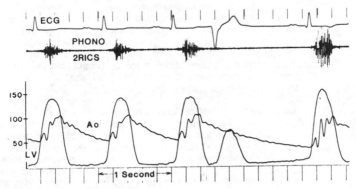

**Figure 12.1   Aortic Stenosis**
The relationship of the pressure gradient to the murmur is demonstrated in the postextrasystolic beat in a patient with aortic stenosis.   The increase in the left ventricular-aortic pressure gradient is matched by an increase in murmur intensity and duration.

An **exception** to this rule occurs when the ventricle with outflow obstruction has an alternate outlet as in the tetralogy of Fallot, in which case a short (or absent) systolic murmur is associated with severe obstruction (or atresia) of the pulmonary outflow tract.

B.   Significant pulmonary stenosis is almost invariably associated with ECG manifestations of right ventricular hypertrophy (RVH).   Therefore, the absence of RVH virtually rules out pulmonary stenosis.   The absence of left ventricular hypertrophy on ECG is less reliable in ruling out aortic stenosis.

C.   The flow disturbance caused by **valvar** stenosis or coarctation usually leads to enlargement, or post-stenotic dilatation, of the portion of the great artery downstream from the stenotic lesion.   An **exception** to this rule occurs in the tetralogy of Fallot because the alternate outflow pathway (aorta) diminishes pulmonary blood flow and therefore turbulence;   low pulmonary blood flow ensues, and the pulmonary artery is small.

D.  Subvalvar and supravalvar stenoses are usually **not** associated with post-stenotic dilatation. One exception is the tetralogy of Fallot with infundibular stenosis and absence, not atresia, of the pulmonary valve leaflets; the main pulmonary artery may have aneurysmal dilatation.

2.  **COMMUNICATIONS** between chambers, great vessels, or great vessels and chambers behave predictably. If the communication is sufficiently large (**nonrestrictive**), it will equalize the pressure in the communicating chambers or great vessels. For example, a ventricular septal defect (VSD) as large as the aortic orifice will equalize the pressures in the right and left ventricles. On the other hand, a small (**restrictive**) VSD will obstruct flow across the defect and will maintain a significant pressure difference between the ventricles.

   A.  Flow across a restrictive **ventricular** septal defect has high velocity because of the pressure drop across the defect (systemic pressure minus normal right ventricular pressure, approximately an 80 mm Hg pressure gradient) and results in velocities comparable to those in severe aortic or pulmonic stenosis. Therefore, there will be a holosystolic murmur in patients with restrictive ventricular septal defects.

   B.  When there is a restrictive communication between the aorta (Ao) and the pulmonary artery (PA) (e.g., a small patent ductus arteriosus), there is a large pressure gradient and resulting increase in flow velocity which phasically increases in systole and decreases in diastole, leading to a **continuous murmur** which reaches a peak in late systole. Similarly, a continuous murmur results from a restrictive communication between the aorta and a right heart chamber (e.g., ruptured sinus of Valsalva aneurysm).

   C.  Conversely, a **nonrestrictive** ventricular septal defect has no pressure drop across the septum and consequently has flow velocities comparable to that of aortic or pulmonary outflow, so that flow through these large defects usually produces little or no murmur.

   D.  Flow through an atrial septal defect occurs throughout the cardiac cycle and is not associated with a pressure drop across the septum. The most common murmur of atrial septal defect is systolic, and results from the two- to fivefold increase in right ventricular outflow which is associated with high velocity and a pressure gradient. A rumbling mid-diastolic murmur that results from the high volume of right ventricular inflow may be heart in the tricuspid area.

   E.  As a general rule, the presence of a systolic or continuous murmur in a patient with congenital heart disease is a

**favorable** sign, since it suggests high flow velocities and a potentially remediable defect. This maxim is particularly helpful in a cyanotic patient, since it implies pulmonary stenosis or atresia and a low pulmonary artery pressure. Alternatively, the **absence** of a significant systolic murmur or the presence of only a diastolic murmur is usually an **ominous** sign, suggesting the lack of either a significant left-to-right shunt or pulmonary stenosis, or the presence of pulmonary hypertension. When pulmonary vascular obliterative changes are present, most forms of definitive or palliative surgery are contraindicated.

F. The **direction** of flow is dictated by the resistance to flow downstream from the chambers communicating through the defect. The resistance to flow downstream can be increased by a stenotic valve, a noncompliant ventricle, or an increase in pulmonary vascular resistance (PVR) or systemic vascular resistance (SVR). It is the relationship of PVR to SVR that determines the direction of flow through a VSD or patent ductus arteriosus (PDA), and the relationship of right ventricular (RV) versus left ventricular (LV) compliance that determines the direction of flow through an ASD.

**Table 12.1**
**Shunt Determination in CHD**

| SITE OF COMMUNICATION | PREDOMINANT SHUNT LEFT TO RIGHT IF: | PREDOMINANT SHUNT RIGHT TO LEFT IF: |
|---|---|---|
| ATRIAL SEPTAL DEFECT | Tricuspid valve normal and RV compliance normal | Tricuspid valve abnormal (stenosis, atresia, severe Ebstein's anomaly) or RV hypertrophied and/or failing due to pulmonary hypertension, stenosis, or chronic volume overload |
| VENTRICULAR SEPTAL DEFECT | VSD restrictive or VSD nonrestrictive with normal RV outflow tract and PVR < SVR | VSD nonrestrictive with RV outflow obstruction (tetralogy of Fallot) or PVR > SVR (Eisenmenger's complex) |
| PATENT DUCTUS ARTERIOSUS | PDA restrictive or PVR < SVR | PDA nonrestrictive and PVR > SVR |

3.   **TRANSPOSITION** (and obligatory shunts due to anomalous connections).

These defects rarely exist in isolation, since most of them are associated with communications or other abnormalities which tend to compensate for the anomaly and contribute to adult survival.

A.   Transposition of the great arteries (TGA), in which the aorta arises from the right ventricle and the pulmonary artery from the left ventricle, is incompatible with survival unless compensated for by associated communications or **ventricular inversion**. Additional **obstruction** of the right ventricular outflow tract also aids in permitting adult survival because it prevents development of pulmonary hypertension.   These are two diagrams of combinations which permit adult survival with TGA.

1)   **TGA with VSD and obstruction of RV outflow.**
Without a VSD, only $O_2$ desaturated blood would circulate through systemic arteries.   Excessive pulmonary blood flow and pulmonary hypertension are moderated by RV outflow obstruction.

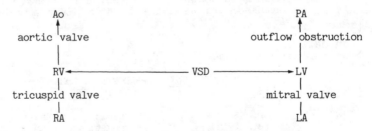

2)   **Corrected TGA** (ventricular inflow inversion).   Ventricular inflow inversion permits the anatomic RV to receive saturated blood from the LA and the LV to receive RA blood.   The systemic arterial blood is therefore fully $O_2$ saturated.

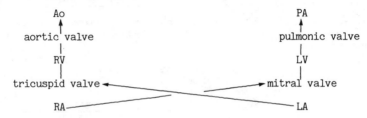

B.   **Anomalous pulmonary venous connection** allows $O_2$ saturated blood to enter the right atrium (RA) or systemic veins, resulting in an obligatory left-to-right shunt and an increase in pulmonary blood flow.

1)   Total anomalous pulmonary venous connection results in all of the pulmonary veins draining into the RA or a systemic vein, and must be associated with an ASD to permit survival. There is a right-to-left shunt at the atrial level and massive pulmonary blood flow.

2)   Partial anomalous pulmonary venous connection (APVC) results in an obligatory venous return from one lobe or the entire right lung into the right heart and an increase in pulmonary blood flow. Partial APVC is often associated with an ASD (usually of the **sinus venosus** type), but survival does not depend on it.

## SUMMARY OF FUNCTIONAL CONSIDERATIONS:

In the absence of transposition, left-to-right shunts increase pulmonary blood flow (PBF) and right-to-left shunts reduce PBF. Most **communications** result in left-to-right shunts unless there is a downstream **obstruction** (e.g., outflow stenosis) or resistance to flow (e.g., hypertrophied RV). **Transposition** of the great arteries always requires compensatory defects for survival.

### COMMON ACYANOTIC FORMS OF CONGENITAL HEART DISEASE PERMITTING ADULT SURVIVAL

| LESION | CLINICAL/LABORATORY FINDINGS |
|---|---|
| A.  OUTFLOW TRACT LESIONS | |
| 1.  Bicuspid Aortic Valve | |
| a.  Without hemodynamic impairment | 1.  Early systolic click, short mid-systolic murmur at 2nd right intercostal space. |
| | 2.  Eccentric closure line of aortic valve on echocardiogram. |
| | 3.  **Significance:** May develop increasingly severe aortic stenosis and/or aortic regurgitation in later life. Prone to infective endocarditis. |

b.  With aortic stenosis

**Figure** 12.2

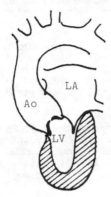

1.  Males/females = 4/1
2.  Delayed carotid upstroke.
3.  Sustained LV lift.
4.  Early systolic click, mid-systolic murmur at R base, transmitted to carotids and apex.
5.  LVH on ECG.
6.  **Significance:**  (See #3 above).  If symptomatic or associated with signifi-cant ECG changes, should be evaluated by Doppler study and/or cardiac catheterization.  Surgery increases survival.

c.  With aortic regurgitation

Note: All forms of discrete LV outflow obstruction share common clinical features: slow pulse upstroke, mid systolic murmur, LVH on ECG, etc.  The differentiating features will be outlined under each lesion.

1.  Bounding pulses, bisfer-iens carotid pulse.
2.  Click, systolic murmur as in AS.
3.  Diastolic blow along left sternal border (LSB).
4.  LVH on ECG
5.  **Significance:**  May be well tolerated for years.  Indications for operative intervention outlined in Chapter 11.

2.  Supravalvar Aortic Stenosis

**Figure** 12.3

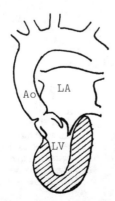

1.  Abnormal facies and dentition with mental retardation ("What, me worry?" - Alfred E. Neumann) common.
2.  Different BP in arms (R > L).
3.  No click.  Mid-systolic murmur at R base, loud $A_2$.
4.  Echo may demonstrate narrow aorta above valve.
5.  **Significance:**  May be fam-ilial.  Cardiac catheter-ization indicated if lesion suspected.

3.  Discrete subvalvar
    aortic atenosis

**Figure 12.4**

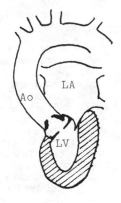

1.  Slow carotid upstroke.
2.  No click.  Mid-systolic
    murmur along LSB.
3.  Soft murmur of AR common.
4.  Echo may demonstrate con-
    striction of LV outflow
    tract and early closure
    of aortic valve.
5.  **Significance:**  May develop
    secondary hypertrophy and
    resemble hypertrophic
    cardiomyopathy.  Cardiac
    catheterization indicated
    if lesion suspected.
    Turbulence in outflow
    tract results in trauma
    to aortic valve leaflets.

4.  Coarctation of
    aorta

**Figure 12.5**

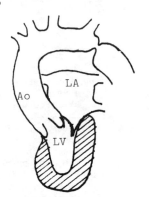

1.  Hypertension in upper ex-
    tremities, slow-rising
    pulses and low BP in
    legs.
2.  Visible collateral
    arteries on back.
3.  Rib notching on chest
    x-ray.
4.  Echo from suprasternal
    notch may demonstrate
    coarctation.
5.  **Significance:**  Often over-
    looked as cause of hyper-
    tension.  Operation best
    in young patients.
    May be managed with anti-
    hypertensive therapy in
    older individuals(5).

Note:   This lesion is often associated with a bicuspid aortic valve.

5.  Hypertrophic
    cardiomyopathy (HCM)
    (See Chapter 13)

**Figure 12.6**

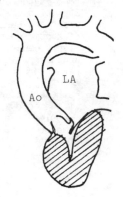

1.  Often familial history of
    heart disease or sudden
    death; patient may be
    asymptomatic or have
    dyspnea, syncope, or chest
    pain.
2.  Brisk carotid upstroke,
    sustained apical impulse.
3.  S4 and loud mid-to-late
    systolic murmur which
    increases with Valsalva.
4.  LVH on ECG--often
    striking.
5.  Echo can be diagnostic
    (see Chapter 4).
6.  **Significance:** Appropri-
    ate therapy (SBE prophy-
    laxis, beta blockers,
    antiarrhythmics, avoid-
    ance of exercise) may
    lower mortality even in
    asymptomatic patients.
    Operation does not lower
    mortality.

6.  Subvalvar pulmonic stenosis

    a.  Rare as isolated lesion
    b.  May coexist with HCM
        or VSD

7.  Valvar pulmonic stenosis

**Figure 12.7**

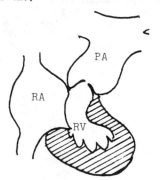

1.  May have round facies.
2.  Prominent jugular venous
    a wave.
3.  RV lift, with systolic
    thrill and murmur at
    upper LSB.  P2 soft
    and late, click may be
    heard.
4.  RVH, RAE on ECG.
5.  Post-stenotic dilatation
    of PA on x-ray.
6.  **Significance:** If no RVH,
    pulmonary stenosis is
    unlikely.  If present,
    cardiac catheterization
    is indicated.  Surgery
    is low risk; good
    results can be antici-
    pated.

8.   Supravalvar pulmonic stenosis

   a.   Usually a result of
        maternal rubella infection
        during pregnancy
   b.   Usually bilateral and
        multiple

B.   LEFT-TO-RIGHT SHUNTS

   1.   Atrial septal defect

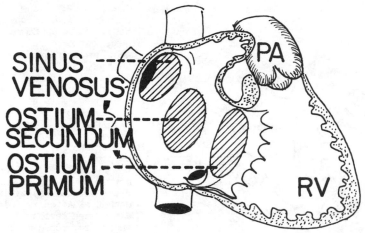

**Figure 12.8**
A right anterior oblique diagram of the right heart chambers
demonstrating the location of the three common types of atrial septal
defects.   **Sinus venosus** defects are in the superior dorsal atrial septum
and are almost invariably associated with partial anomalous pulmonary
venous drainage into the right atrium.   **Ostium secundum** defects result
from excessive resorption of the embryologic septum primum; these defects
are usually large and may be fenestrated.   **Ostium primum** defects result
from failure of fusion of the embryologic endocardial cushion and septum
primum, resulting in an inferior defect associated with mitral and
tricuspid valve deformities (cleft septal leaflets with or without
regurgitation).

a. Ostium secundum

1. Most common ASD, females/males = 2/1.
2. Mitral prolapse present in 1/3.
3. Often not symptomatic until 4th to 6th decade.
4. RV and PA lift; fixed split S2, with mid-systolic murmur. Ejection click common.
5. Enlarged right heart and pulmonary plethora on chest x-ray; "hilar dance" on fluoroscopy.
6. Shunt can be confirmed and quantitated by radio-nuclide angiography.
7. RSR' or RSR'S' in V1 common, with normal or right axis. P-R may be prolonged. Atrial fibrillation in older patients.
8. **Significance:** Since lesion has low-risk repair and may become inoperable in later life (as RV fails and pulmonary hypertension develops, R-L shunt occurs) cardiac catheterization is indicated when lesion is suspected. Operation is indicated if heart enlarged and PBF:SBF is >2:1. SBE prophylaxis usually not required (unless mitral prolapse murmur present).

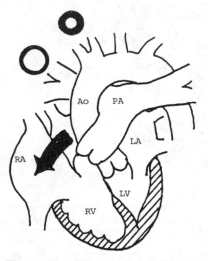

**Figure 12.9 Atrial Septal Defect**
In this depiction of a young patient with an ASD, there is a left-to-right shunt because the RV compliance (distensibility) is greater than that of the LV. With a large (nonrestrictive) ASD, the pressures in the atria are equal and the flow follows the line of least resistance. The pulmonary vascular resistance (thin circle adjacent to the right pulmonary artery) is low, permitting high flow without elevation of the pulmonary artery pressure. The right heart chambers and PA are dilated to accommodate the high flow (volume overload).

Note: All types of ASD share common features as outlined under ostium secundum. Differentiating features will be noted under other defects.

b. Sinus venosus

1. Often associated with partial anomalous pulmonary venous connection.
2. **Significance:** Low-risk surgery can close defect and reroute anomalous pulmonary veins.

c. Ostium primum

1. Left and superior axis deviation of ECG plus RSR'S' highly suggestive of diagnosis.
2. Mitral regurgitant murmur may be present.
3. Surgery carries slight risk of acquired heart block. Mitral valve may require repair, rarely replacement.

d. Miscellaneous

1. Defects may be multiple (ostium primum + secundum), or entire septum may be absent ("single atrium").
2. Various eponyms are associated with ASD complexes:
   a. Holt-Oram syndrome: Hypoplastic thumb + ostium secundum ASD.
   b. Ellis-van Creveld syndrome: Polydactyly + single atrium.
   c. Lutembacher's syndrome: Mitral stenosis (probably rheumatic) + ASD.

2. Ventricular septal
defects

a.  Maladie de Roger

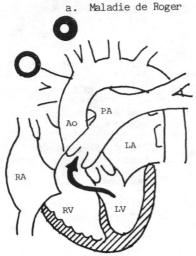

1.  Small VSD.
2.  Left parasternal thrill
    with loud holosystolic
    murmur at 4 left inter-
    costal space.
3.  Chest x-ray and ECG may be
    normal.
4.  Cardiac catheterization
    unnecessary.  Lesion can
    be confirmed by Doppler
    study.
5.  **Significance:**  Clinical
    course usually benign(4).
    SBE prophylaxis is
    indicated.

**Figure 12.10  Maladie de Roger**
A small (restrictive) ventricular septal defect that serves to limit the
magnitude of the left-to-right shunt and does not increase the right heart
pressure significantly.   The pulmonary vascular resistance (indicated by
the thin circle opposite the right pulmonary artery) is normal.

b.  Large VSD with
    L-R shunt

1.  Relatively rare in adults
    (most large VSDs develop
    pulmonary hypertension in
    childhood).
2.  Heart enlarged with
    active RV and LV. Holo-
    systolic murmur at lower
    left sternal border.
    S2 split, not fixed.
3.  Lesion can be confirmed
    by Doppler study.
4.  Radionuclide shunt study
    will confirm and quan-
    titate shunt.
5.  **Significance:**  May be
    associated with aortic
    regurgitation due to loss
    of support of valve.

Cardiac catheterization is indicated, and surgery indicated if large L-R shunt confirmed and PVR not greatly increased.

Note: Septal defects can be supracristal or infra-cristal relative to the crista supraventricularis.

3. Patent ductus arteriosus

1. Females/males = 2/1.
2. Continuous murmur peaking at S2, best heard in left infraclavicular area.
3. If shunt large, heart will be enlarged and pulmonary vascularity increased.
4. **Significance:** Complete restoration to normal is possible with low-risk surgery in young patients. In older patients, risk increases due to friability of ductus and aortic isthmus. Rarely, ductus may recur if ligated and not divided.

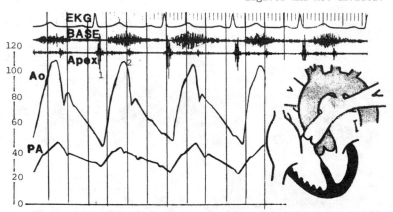

**Figure 12.11 Patent ductus arteriosus**
The Ao pressure is higher than the PA pressure throughout the cardiac cycle, which results in pulsatile continuous flow and a murmur at the base which spills through and obscures the second heart sound(2). The PA pressure is elevated to 50/25 because of the high flow state (PBF:SBF = 5:1), but the pulmonary vascular resistance is normal.

4.  Other causes of "continuous murmurs" which may simulate PDA in acyanotic patients

   a.  Anomalous origin of left coronary artery from pulmonary artery
   b.  Coronary-cameral fistulae (coronary artery to cardiac chamber)
   c.  Pulmonary arterio-venous (AV) fistulae
   d.  Congenital or acquired AV fistulae
   e.  VSD with aortic regurgitation
   f.  Ruptured sinus of Valsalva aneurysms (aorta to right heart chamber)
   g.  Venous hum
   h.  Coarctation of aorta
   i.  Pulmonary artery branch stenoses

C.  Congenital Complete Heart Block

1.  May be familial.
2.  Heart rate of < 50, pulse bounding, jugular venous cannon a waves, variable S1
3.  Systolic (flow) murmur along LSB, often mistaken for VSD.
4.  High mortality in first year of life, usually stable course in first 3-4 decades.

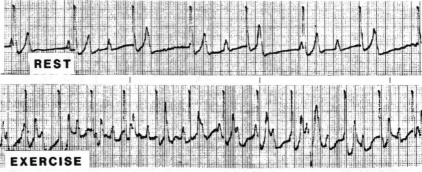

**Figure 12.12  Congenital Complete Heart Block.** An electrocardiographic rhythm strip at rest demonstrates dissociated atrial and ventricular complexes with a ventricular rate of 43. With exercise, the ventricular rate is 80.

D. Corrected transposition of great arteries

1. May have no associated lesions, but following are commonly found:
   a. Heart block.
   b. Abnormal left AV valve (Ebstein's deformity, with left AV valve regurgitation).
   c. VSD with or without subpulmonic stenosis.
   d. Dextrocardia.

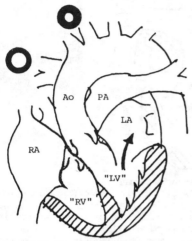

**Figure 12.13 Corrected Transposition of the Great Arteries**
The congenital "correction" consists of inversion of the inflow tracts of the two ventricles, so that the trabecular RV with its tricuspid valve links up with the LA and its pulmonary venous (oxygenated) blood, and the LV with its bicuspid (mitral) valve receives RA blood. Thus, the "RV" which pumps blood to the PA is morphologically an LV, and the Ao receives blood from an "LV" which has the architecture of an RV. Left AV valve incompetence is common (arrow). Corrected transposition may be associated with ventricular septal defect and subpulmonic stenosis (not shown), and if the subpulmonic stenosis is sufficiently severe, cyanosis may result.

Corrected transposition is almost invariably a **levo** transposition, in which the aorta is to the left of the pulmonary artery as a result of the embryonic bulboventricular loop bending to the left, instead of the normal rightward anterior loop. A leftward loop would be concordant with the rest of the body in **situs inversus** in which dextrocardia would be "normal," but when it occurs in **situs solitus** (normal body position), there is often a discordant dextrocardia or dextroposition. Therefore, a **levo** transposition can be anticipated when the heart is in the right thorax, and corrected transposition can be suspected when there is dextrocardia with minimal disability.

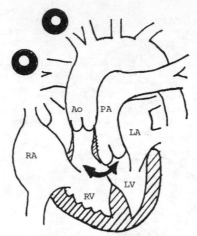

**Figure 12.14  Transposition of the Great Arteries**
This invariably cyanotic condition is illustrated here for comparison
with corrected transposition.  There is an obligatory desaturation of
the Ao blood, since the RV receives systemic venous blood and is in
continuity with the Ao.  Survival depends on admixture, in this example
at ventricular level.  Because the pulmonary vascular bed is not
protected by outflow tract stenosis in this example, the pulmonary
vascular resistance is elevated (thickened circle).  The aorta is to the
right of the pulmonary artery.

**COMMON CYANOTIC FORMS OF CONGENITAL
HEART DISEASE PERMITTING ADULT SURVIVAL**

A.  **SEPTAL DEFECTS WITH DOWN-
    STREAM RESISTANCE**

1.  Tetralogy of Fallot

    a.  Nonrestrictive VSD
    b.  RV outflow obstruction
    c.  RV hypertrophy
    d.  "Overriding aorta"

1.  Severity of outflow
    stenosis will determine
    degree of cyanosis.
2.  History of cyanosis at
    birth,cyanotic spells, and
    squatting in childhood.
3.  Exercise increases degree
    of cyanosis.
4.  Cyanosis (rest or with
    exercise), clubbing,
    single S2, outflow
    stenosis murmur.
5.  ECG:  RVH or biventricular
    hypertrophy.

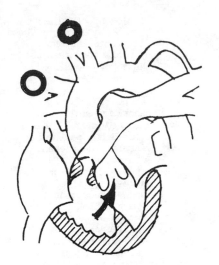

6. X-ray: Boot-shaped heart (small pulmonary artery, apex tipped up).
7. Hematocrit will reflect mean daily level of arterial desaturation unless patient is iron depleted.
8. Many adults with tetralogy of Fallot have had palliative systemic pulmonary shunts created. If patent, a continuous murmur will be heard.
9. **Significance:** Potentially correctable in most cases. Cardiac catheterization and consideration of surgery indicated in all suspected cases.

**Figure 12.15 Tetralogy of Fallot (with Blalock-Taussig Shunt)**
There is a large nonrestrictive ventricular septal defect and obstruction to outflow of the RV at two levels: infundibular and valvar. The PA is underdeveloped and the RV is hypertrophic because it generates systemic pressure. There is a right-to-left shunt (arrow) directly from the RV into the Ao because the resistance to aortic outflow is less than through the stenotic RV outflow tract. A palliative left Blalock-Taussig shunt (subclavian-PA anastomosis), which increases the quantity of oxygenated blood entering the LV and therefore raises the Ao blood oxygenation, is shown. The normal pulmonary vascular resistance is indicated by the thin circle adjacent to the right pulmonary artery.

Note: If the right ventricular outflow tract or the main pulmonary artery is atretic (absent or completely interrupted), the pulmonary arteries derive their blood from bronchial collaterals. This severe form of tetralogy is often called a "type IV truncus arteriosus." In this situation, the only murmurs heard are the continuous murmurs from the systemic-pulmonary collaterals. Although the entire right ventricular outflow traverses the VSD into the aorta, this flow produces no murmur because it is a nonrestrictive defect.

2.  Eisenmenger Complex
    (large VSD with
    pulmonary hypertension)

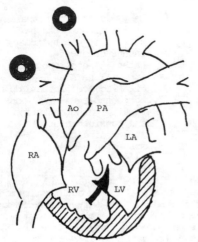

1.  Developent of pulmonary
    hypertension in childhood
    diminishes L-R shunt,
    cyanosis increases as
    shunt reverses (R-L).
2.  Dyspnea on exertion but
    no LV failure.
3.  Hemoptysis.
4.  Heart size small because of
    balanced shunt.  Main PA
    dilated but peripheral
    vessels constricted.
5.  On exam, RV and PA
    impulse, single or
    narrowly split S2,
    murmur of pulmonary
    regurgitation (no VSD
    murmur.
6.  **Significance:** "Fixed"
    high pulmonary vascular
    resistance precludes
    cardiac surgical correc-
    tion, but with careful
    medical management (treat-
    ment of arrhythmias,
    phlebotomy for hematocrit
    over 60%, etc.) reason-
    able longevity possible.

**Figure 12.16  Eisenmenger Complex**
There is a large nonrestrictive VSD and the pulmonary vascular bed is
unprotected from the resulting systemic RV pressure.  The shunt (arrow)
is right to left because the pulmonary arteriolar resistance (thick
circle) exceeds systemic vascular resistance.  The pulmonary
hypertension is irreversible and closure of the VSD would be fatal.

3.  "Eisenmenger Reaction"
    (ASD or PDA with
    pulmonary hypertension)

    a.  ASD with reversed shunt

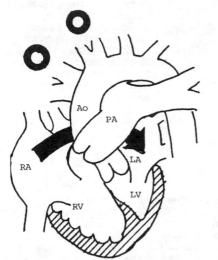

1.  A late complication of
    large ASD, usually after
    5th decade.  The shunt
    reverses when RV fails
    and/or pulmonary vascular
    resistance increases.
2.  Right heart and pulmonary
    arteries  enlarged because
    of large intracardiac
    shunt for 3-4 decades.
3.  RV lift, widely split S2,
    murmur of tricuspid, and/
    or pulmonic regurgitation.
4.  ECG:  RBBB or rsR',
    atrial fibrillation
    common.
5.  **Significance:**  Cardiac
    catheterization indicated
    to assess pulmonary vas-
    cular resistance.
    Surgical closure of ASD
    is possible if resistance
    is less than 5 units or
    decreases markedly with
    oxygen breathing.

**Figure 12.17  Atrial Septal Defect with Reversed Shunt**
The Eisenmenger reaction results from many years of exposure to high
pulmonary blood flow which leads to dilated, hypertrophic, failing RV
which becomes less receptive to atrial inflow than the LV.   The pulmonary
vascular resistance (thickened circle) rarely exceeds systemic vascular
resistance with ASD, and its effect on the shunt is indirect; the elevated
pressure leads to RV hypertrophy and eventually a decreased ejection
fraction.  The resulting thickened RV with a large end-systolic volume
resists diastolic filling.

b.  Patent ductus

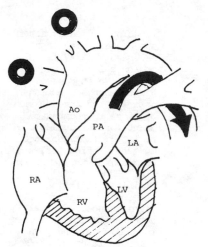

1.  Size of PDA is large and pulmonary hypertension is usually established early in life.
2.  Reversed flow through PDA is extracardiac, so heart is not enlarged.
3.  On exam, feet are cyanotic and clubbed, fingers acyanotic.  No murmur, or murmur of pulmonary regurgitation.
4.  **Significance:** Inoperable, but patients may do quite well with conservative management(1).

**Figure 12.18  Patent Ductus with Shunt Reversal**
There is a large nonrestrictive ductus which results in equalization of pressures in the Ao and PA.  When the pulmonary vascular resistance exceeds systemic resistance, there is shunt reversal, with desaturated blood entering the descending thoracic aorta (arrow) and causing cyanosis of the lower extremities (differential cyanosis).

"Reversed differential cyanosis," or blue fingers and pink toes, can be seen when there is transposition of the great arteries (TGA) with a PDA and pulmonary hypertension.

A common misconception is that differential cyanosis and reversed differential cyanosis can result from a PDA in combination with a coarctation of the aorta.  It should be noted that the aortic pressure downstream from a coarctation is at **systemic** level (mean pressure 70-90 mm Hg) so that it would be necessary to have pulmonary hypertension for right-to-left shunting through a PDA, with or without a coarctation.

4. Ebstein's Anomaly of the Tricuspid Valve

1. Abnormally placed and deformed tricuspid valve.
2. Hypoplastic right ventricle.
3. Frequently associated with patent foramen ovale.
4. Degree of cyanosis dependent on degree of inadequacy of tricuspid valve (obstruction and/or regurgitation) and abnormal RV function.
5. Auscultation often reveals multiple heart sounds: split S1("sail sound" of late tricuspid closure), split S2(RBBB), S3, and S4. Murmurs may be present in systole (tricuspid regurgitation), diastole, or presystole.
6. ECG: Wide, bizarre RSR' complex in V1. Right atrial enlargement. Atrial fibrillation common.
7. Associated with Wolff-Parkinson-White syndrome.
8. X-ray: Enlarged heart, especially right atrium, with decreased pulmonary vascularity.
9. Echocardiography: Diagnostic enlargement of anterior tricuspid leaflet, displaced septal leaflet, and delayed closure of anterior leaflet.
10. **Significance:** May present with arrhythmias in middle age.

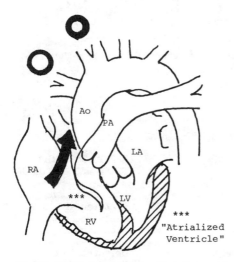

**Figure 12.19 Ebstein's Anomaly**
The tricuspid valve is deformed and the RV walls are hypoplastic. A patent foramen ovale permits right-to-left shunting (arrow) and causes variable cyanosis. The pulmonary arteriolar resistance is normal. The displaced tricuspid valve creates an "atrialized ventricular chamber" (***) that is upstream of the tricuspid valve but within the RV walls. The tricuspid valve is often incompetent.

OPERATIVE INTERVENTIONS IN CONGENITAL HEART DISEASE

Operations for congenital heart defects can be divided into **palliative** or **definitive** categories. Although terms such as "total correction" and "curative" are used as synonyms for definitive procedures, these terms (with rare exceptions) reflect unwarranted optimism. Two procedures that can be truly curative (in that the heart can be completely normal afterwards) are ligation with division of a small patent ductus and suture closure of an atrial septal defect in childhood. All other procedures entail certain compromises such as ventriculotomy and the use of prosthetic materials or construction of conduits, or may leave residual functional abnormalities such as chamber enlargement, impaired contractility, conduction defect, outflow obstruction, valvar regurgitation, or persistent or new murmurs.

**Palliative** operations are usually associated with lower risk than definitive procedures, and thus can be used as temporizing measures that permit survival of critically ill patients until a more definitive intervention can be undertaken. Most palliative procedures actually add new defects and therefore may increase the complexity of the later definitive repair. However, this theoretical disadvantage is counterbalanced by the improved functional status and maturity of the patient.

Tables 12.2 and 12.3 define palliative and definitive procedures and the clinical indications for their use.

**TABLE 12.2**

**PALLIATIVE PROCEDURES IN CONGENITAL HEART DISEASE**

| PROCEDURES | PURPOSE | DEFECTS FOR WHICH PROCEDURES ARE USED |
|---|---|---|
| *1. Pulmonary artery banding | Decreases excessive pulmonary blood flow to prevent pulmonary hypertension | Nonrestrictive ventricular septal defects with normal great vessel orientation or transposition of the great vessels |

**TABLE** 12.2 (continued)

| | | |
|---|---|---|
| *2. Creation of atrial septal defect<br>  A. **RASHKIND:**<br>    Catheter balloon<br>    or blade septostomy<br>  B. **BLALOCK-HANLON:**<br>    Closed heart<br>    surgical excision<br>    of posterior<br>    interatrial septum | Brings oxygenated blood into right atrium, right ventricle, and aorta | Transposition of the great arteries |
| 3. Systemic--pulmonary artery anastomosis<br> *A. **BLALOCK-TAUSSIG:**<br>    Subclavian-pulmonary artery anastomosis (end to side) | Increases pulmonary blood flow and oxygenation of aortic blood | Cyanotic CHD with decreased pulmonary blood flow and low pulmonary artery pressure:<br>- tetralogy of Fallot<br>- pulmonary atresia<br>- tricuspid atresia |

  *B. **POTTS:**
    Descending aorta-left
    pulmonary artery anastomosis
    (side to side)
  *C. **WATERSTON-COOLEY:**
    Ascending aorta-right pulmonary artery
    (side to side)

Note: The Potts and Waterston-Cooley procedures have theoretical advantages over the Blalock-Taussig shunt: greater flow, better systemic oxygenation, and avoidance of sacrificing the subclavian artery. In contrast, the Blalock-Taussig anastomoses may become progressively restrictive as the patient grows, leading to decreasing flow, declining systemic oxygenation, and a rising hematocrit. However, the ease of ablating the subclavian-pulmonary anastomosis at the time of definitive repair compared to the technical complexity of closing a Potts or Waterston-Cooley shunt has led to a greater use of the original "blue baby operation."

4. Right ventricular bypass
   *A. Partial. **GLENN:**
   Superior cava to right
   pulmonary artery
   anastomosis (end to
   end)

   Increases pul-
   monary blood
   flow and oxygen-
   ation of aortic
   blood

   Tricuspid
   atresia

5. Venous return inversion
   *A. Partial. **BAFFES:**
   Right pulmonary vein-
   right atrial anasto-
   mosis

   Increases oxygen-
   ation of RA and
   aortic blood,
   improves mixing

   Transposition
   of great
   arteries

   B. Complete "atrial
   switch." **PALLIATIVE
   MUSTARD/SENNING:**
   Excision of atrial
   septum, baffle
   inserted to route
   pulmonary venous blood
   through tricuspid
   valve to RV, caval
   blood through mitral
   valve to LV (VSD
   not repaired)

   Brings oxygenated
   blood to RA and
   RV to improve
   aortic oxygen
   saturation

   Transposition
   of great
   arteries with
   VDS and
   pulmonary
   hypertension
   (Eisenmenger
   transposition)

*These procedures do not require cardiopulmonary bypass.

**TABLE 12.3**

**DEFINITIVE OPERATIVE TREATMENT OF COMPLEX CONGENITAL HEART DISEASE**

Definitive repair is defined as procedures that completely separate right
heart and left heart circuits resulting in an "in series circuit."

| PROCEDURES | DEFECTS FOR WHICH PROCEDURES ARE USED |
|---|---|
| 1. Intracardiac repair: Closure of VSD by patch, enlargement of outflow tract by resection, or resection plus patch; with DORV or transposition, septal defect patch is fashioned to connect LV and aorta. | Tetralogy of Fallot<br><br>Double outlet right ventricle (DORV) with pulmonic stenosis<br><br>Transposition (when combined with Rastelli--see below) |

TABLE 12.3 (continued)

2. **RASTELLI:**
   Extracardiac conduit from right ventricle to pulmonary artery, with or without valve

   Pulmonary atresia with ASD or VSD; DORV or transposition of great arteries (when combined with internal tunnel patch from left ventricle to aorta)

3. "Atrial switch":
   **MUSTARD/SENNING:**
   Excision of atrial septum with creation of a baffle-septum that routes all of pulmonary venous return through tricuspid valve to RV and caval blood through mitral valve to LV.  Closure of VSD and/or repair of pulmonic stenosis if present

   Transposition of great arteries without pulmonary hypertension

4. "Arterial switch":
   Aorta and pulmonary arteries are separated from their semilunar valves and translocated to alignment with appropriate ventricle; coronary arteries are anastomosed (usually via grafts) to the translocated aorta

   Transposition of the great arteries without pulmonary hypertension and good left ventricular function

5. **FONTAN:**
   Right atrium to pulmonary artery anastomosis with oversewing of tricuspid and/or pulmonic valve

   Tricuspid atresia, single ventricle with pulmonic stenosis or atresia

## REFERENCES

1. Campbell M:  Natural history of persistent ductus arteriosus.  Br Heart J 30:4-13, 1968.

2. Coles JG, Garely NF, Butteglien JB:  Congenital heart disease in the adult.  Arch Surg 89:130-134, 1964.

3. Cooley DA, Hallman GL, Hammam AS:  Congenital cardiovascular anomalies in adults.  Result of surgical treatment in 167 patients over 35.  Am J Cardiol 17:303-309, 1966.

4. Corone P, Doyon F, Gauden S, et al.:  Natural history of ventricular septal defect.  A study involving 790 cases.  Circulation 55:908-915, 1977.

5. Liberthson RR, Pennington DG, Jacobs ML, et al.:  Coarctation of the aorta:  Review of 234 patients and clarification of management problems.  Am J Cardiol 43:835-840, 1979.

6. Perloff JK:  The Clinical Recognition of Congenital Heart Disease.  Philadelphia, W.B Saunders Co., 1983.

7. Robert WC:  Congenital Heart Disease in Adults.  Philadelphia, F.A. Davis Co., 1986.

8. Ross EA, Perloff JK, Danovitch GM, et al.:  Renal function and urate metabolism in late survivors with cyanotic congenital heart disease.  Circulation 73:396-400, 1986.

# Chapter 13

# The Cardiomyopathies

## CLASSIFICATION

A specific etiology or associated disease will be found in fewer than 10% of patients ultimately found to have a cardiomyopathy. Thus, the **"primary" cardiomyopathies (those of unknown etiology) are far more common than the "secondary" cardiomyopathies (those of known etiology or associated with a systemic disease which involves the heart as part of a recognized disease process).** The cardiomyopathies may be classified according to etiology or they may be separated into a broad and potentially more useful **descriptive classification in terms of** management by grouping them according to the nature of the **hemodynamic fault** into three different categories: 1) dilated or congestive, 2) hypertrophic, and 3) restrictive.

## DILATED CARDIOMYOPATHY

This group is **characterized by poor myocardial systolic function.** Left ventricular contractility is diminished, leading to a decrease in cardiac output and increased end-systolic and end-diastolic ventricular volumes and pressures. Cardiomegaly resulting more from dilatation than hypertrophy is invariably present.

The idiopathic or primary dilated cardiomyopathies are included within this group(1). **Systemic diseases which may involve the heart and produce a dilated cardiomyopathy** as part of a recognized disease process include the following:

1. **Connective Tissue Diseases.** Systemic lupus erythematosus, scleroderma, polyarteritis nodosa, polymyositis.

2. **Neuromuscular Disorders.** The muscular dystrophies, Friedrich's ataxia, peroneal muscular atrophy.

3. **Infection.** Viral (Coxsackie A and B), parasitic (Chagas' disease, trichinosis, toxoplasmosis). Bacterial infections more commonly produce an acute myocarditis.

4. **Endocrine/Metabolic Disorders.** Thyrotoxicosis, myxedema, beri-beri, starvation, glycogen storage diseases, mucopolysaccharidosis.

5. **Myocardial "Toxins."** Emetine, cobalt, alcohol, daunorubicin (Adriamycin).

6. **Infiltrative.** Amyloidosis, sarcoidosis, hemochromatosis.

7. **Miscellaneous.** Postpartum cardiomyopathy.

CLINICAL PROFILE:

As predicted from the hemodynamic fault, **patients most commonly present with signs and symptoms of congestive heart failure**(2) (see Chapter 10). In addition, it is not uncommon for the patient to present with signs of a myocardial, cerebral, renal, or mesenteric infarction or a pulseless, blue extremity due to an **embolus from a mural thrombus**. **Sudden death** is frequent in patients with a dilated cardiomyopathy, especially if associated with neuromuscular disorders or sarcoidosis, disorders characterized by a high frequency of conduction system disease.

**Murmurs** are frequently heard during cardiac auscultation and are not themselves indicative of primary valvular disease. A holosystolic mitral or tricuspid regurgitation murmur is very common and is due to ventricular dilatation and resultant lateral displacement of the papillary muscles which inhibits leaflet coaptation(3). Annular dilatation does not occur to a significant degree(4). Occasionally, an apical "diastolic rumble" may also be heard and is due either to increased early diastolic atrioventricular flow, the result of mitral regurgitation, or a loud summation gallop(5).

The **chest x-ray** most commonly shows cardiomegaly and evidence of pulmonary venous and arterial hypertension.

The **electrocardiogram** is almost always abnormal. In addition to evidence of ventricular and atrial enlargement, Q or QS waves and poor R wave progression across the anterior precordial leads are frequently seen. AV nodal and intraventricular conduction defects and arrhythmias, particularly atrial fibrillation and premature ventricular depolarizations, are common associated findings. Left bundle branch block is common in dilated cardiomyopathy.

The characteristic **echocardiographic** findings (Chapter 4, Figure 4.8) in a patient with a congestive cardiomyopathy reflect poor contractile function: decreased ejection fraction (increased E-point septal separation), decreased velocity of circumferential fiber shortening, increased end-systolic and end-diastolic volumes, left ventricular and left atrial chamber enlargement, and early rapid diastolic motion of the mitral valve (suggesting rapid, early diastolic left ventricular filling and mitral regurgitation).

## MANAGEMENT:

The goal of therapy is to alleviate the symptomatic manifestations of congestive heart failure (see Chapter 10).  Additional interventions in the case of a secondary cardiomyopathy will be dictated by the underlying disease, such as complete abstinence in the case of alcoholic cardiomyopathy.

## HYPERTROPHIC CARDIOMYOPATHY

Within the context of this discussion, hypertrophic cardiomyopathy (HCM) refers to idiopathic or primary cardiac hypertrophy--increased ventricular muscle mass without associated increase in cavity size-- characterized anatomically by asymmetric hypertrophy of the septum.   The disorder may be familial (the majority have autosomal dominant transmission) or sporadic.  This disorder has also been called hyper- trophic obstructive cardiomyopathy (HOCM), idiopathic hypertrophic subaortic stenosis (IHSS), and muscular subaortic stenosis (MSS), to name a few.  The pathophysiologic mechanism(s) underlying the observed clinical and hemodynamic findings remains an area of active investigation and debate(6).

Hemodynamically, **hypertrophic cardiomyopathy is characterized by poor diastolic function of the left ventricle due to reduced compliance.** The decrease in compliance is reflected in an increased left ventricular (LV) end-diastolic pressure and impedance to diastolic filling. Systolic function is maintained (normal cardiac output, ejection fraction, and end-diastolic volume)(7).   A systolic pressure gradient between the body of the left ventricle and the outflow tract may be recorded in some patients at rest or following provocation (i.e., exercise, Valsalva maneuver, or isoproterenol infusion) (Figure 13.1). Proposed explanations for this gradient include: 1) dynamic outflow obstruction by the hypertrophied septum, 2) outflow obstruction by the anterior leaflet of the mitral valve during systole, and 3) forceful, exaggerated LV contraction with late systolic isometric contraction(6). The variability of the gradient and the fact that the left ventricle ejects nearly its entire volume during the first half of systole suggests that true obstruction or impediment to outflow does not occur.  The presence of symptoms and the higher apparent death rate in symptomatic patients **without** pressure gradients renders the significance of the pressure gradient unclear.

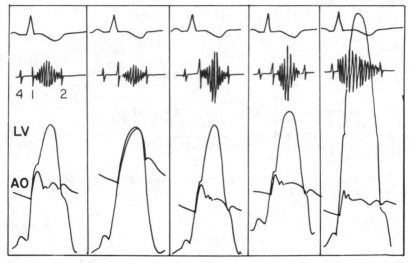

**CONTROL PRESSOR DILATOR VALSALVA POST ECTOPIC**

**Figure 13.1   Pressure Gradients in HCM**

Variable pressure gradients between the left ventricular cavity (LV) and the aorta (Ao) may be recorded during cardiac catheterization of a patient with HCM. In this figure, Ao and LV pressure recordings and a phonocardiogram demonstrate characteristic hemodynamic and auscultatory findings in HCM. The LV-Ao pressure gradient may be present at rest (control) as shown here, may appear spontaneously during the course of the hemodynamic study, or may manifest itself only after provocation. Interventions that decrease ventricular filling (Valsalva maneuver), lower arterial resistance (vasodilators such as amyl nitrate), or increase the force of ventricular contraction (isoproterenol or postectopic beat) may provoke the appearance of a gradient and systolic murmur not present at rest or enhance an existing LV-Ao gradient and systolic murmur as shown here. Increasing the impedance to left ventricular ejection using a vasopressor agent will decrease the magnitude of the gradient. Provocation of a pressure gradient in a patient without other evidence of HCM should not be considered diagnostic of HCM because such a gradient can be produced in normal hearts and in patients with other cardiac conditions(7).

## CLINICAL PROFILE:

Dyspnea on exertion, chest pain which may be anginal in character, palpitations, and/or syncope are the **major symptoms** in patients with hypertrophic cardiomyopathy(7). A family history of sudden death or "heart failure" is not uncommon. This disease may present as sudden death, particularly in younger patients during or after exercise.

**Physical examination** reveals large dominant "a" waves in the jugular venous pulse and a jerky carotid pulse or "pulsus bisfierens." A sustained late systolic left ventricular impulse preceded by a presystolic thrust is noted on palpation of the precordium. A variable mid-to-late systolic murmur and a fourth heart sound may be heard at the apex and left sternal border. The intensity of the systolic murmur is increased by standing and during the strain phase of the Valsalva maneuver(7).

The **chest x-ray** is usually normal. Left ventricular and left atrial hypertrophy are frequently but not always noted on **the electrocardiogram**. Small Q waves in leads V4 through V6 and an R/S ratio in V1 greater than 0.2 are suggestive of hypertrophic cardiomyopathy(8). Less frequently, prominent Q waves in II, III, and aVF are seen and are presumed to result from hypertrophy of the upper septum.

On the **echocardiogram,** an increase in the thickness of the interventricular septum with a lesser increase in the thickness of the LV posterior basal wall is seen (septum to posterior wall thickness ratio of greater than 1.3 -- a reflection of asymmetric septal hypertrophy [ASH]). Additional echocardiographic features include(9): decreased systolic thickening of the septum, systolic anterior motion (SAM) of the anterior leaflet of the mitral valve, decreased E to F slope of the mitral valve, a normal or reduced LV end-diastolic dimension, and mid-systolic closure of the aortic valve (Chapter 4, Figure 4.9). It should be noted that **asymmetric septal hypertrophy on the echocardiogram is not pathognomonic of hypertrophic cardiomyopathy** and has been observed in a number of other conditions: systemic arterial hypertension, valvular aortic stenosis, in healthy athletes, following insertion of prosthetic aortic valves, after inferior myocardial infarction, and in hypothyroid heart disease.

## MANAGEMENT:

The clinical course of patients with hypertrophic cardiomyopathy is extremely variable(10) and not clearly related to the measured systolic pressure gradient. There are limited data available to suggest that medical or surgical therapy alters the course of the disease or the incidence of sudden death.

**Beta-adrenergic** blockade remains the mainstay of therapy and is most useful in alleviating the chest pain associated with this disease. The primary rationale for beta blockade therapy is based on the premise that prevention of exercise tachycardia aids in ventricular filling and reduces the oxygen demands of the ventricle.  Additional benefits are the antiarrhythmic effects of propranolol and the possible blocking of the "hypertrophying" influence of circulating catecholamines.  One clinical study has suggested that daily doses in excess of 320 mg of propranolol will lessen the anticipated annual mortality of 3.6% to less than 1%(11).

**Calcium-blocking agents** (i.e., verapamil) have also been used in selected patients and have been found to alleviate symptoms.  The rationale for their use is based upon their demonstrated effects on myocardial contractility (a decrease in contractility improves the $O_2$ supply/demand ratio)(12,13).  However, verapamil may cause serious hemodynamic complications and should be used cautiously in selected patients(14).

Rapid or unexpected deterioration is commonly associated with the onset of arrhythmias, especially atrial fibrillation, and thus requires aggressive management(7,9).

## RESTRICTIVE CARDIOMYOPATHY

This group is **characterized by varying degrees of systolic and diastolic ventricular dysfunction**(15).  Overall cardiac mass is increased due to myocardial thickening (fibrosis or infiltration) but there is usually only a modest increase in ventricular cavity size.  The major hemodynamic fault is a decrease in ventricular compliance which produces a distinctive early diastolic "dip and plateau" configuration of right and left ventricular pressures.  However, the left ventricular end-diastolic pressure characteristically is higher than right ventricular end-diastolic pressure and serves to distinguish a restrictive cardiomyopathy from constrictive pericarditis(16) (see Chapter 14).  Ventricular end-diastolic volume is usually normal or decreased.  Cardiac output may be normal or decreased, depending upon the extent of replacement of contractile myocardium and the limitation to ventricular filling.

A restrictive cardiomyopathy may be present in the absence of demonstrable systemic disease or cause (idiopathic) or it may occur in association with a known systemic disease process(2).

1. **Amyloidosis.**  Clinically significant cardiac involvement can occur in patients with primary amyloidosis.  Biopsy of the rectal mucosa, skin and/or gingiva may be of value in establishing the diagnosis.  Endomyocardial biopsy may often establish the diagnosis of amyloidosis.  Two-dimensional echocardiography will show thickened ventricular walls and a characteristic "scintillating" pattern of the myocardium(17,18).

2. **Hemochromatosis.**  Significant cardiac involvement occurs in 30% of patients with hemochromatosis and is more commonly encountered in males.  Cardiac involvement more commonly produces a dilated cardiomyopathy.

3. **Sarcoidosis.** The true incidence of "sarcoid cardiomyopathy" is unknown and heart failure in a patient with sarcoid is most commonly due to pulmonary hypertension and cor pulmonale(19). In patients with cardiac sarcoidosis, death is more likely to be due to an arrhythmia than it is to progressive heart failure.

4. **Progressive Systemic Sclerosis (Scleroderma).** Cardiac involvement is second only to renal disease as a cause of death.

5. **Metastatic Malignancy.** Often clinically silent, but metastatic disease to the myocardium has been reported to occur in 5 to 10% of all autopsies in patients with malignant disease.

6. **Glycogen Storage Disease.**

7. **Endomyocardiopathy with Eosinophilia** (hypereosinophilic syndrome).

## CLINICAL PROFILE:

**Patients may present with signs and symptoms of congestive heart failure.** Usually symptoms relate to the systemic disease which causes not only myocardial infiltration but involvement of other organs as well.

**Physical findings may mimic those of constrictive pericarditis** in that a rapid "y" descent of the jugular venous pulse, Kussmaul's sign, and pulsus paradoxus can be noted in patients with restrictive cardiomyopathies. **Cardiac auscultation** usually reveals a third and fourth heart sound and murmurs of mitral and tricuspid regurgitation may be heard. **Chest x-ray** usually shows a normal or slightly enlarged cardiac silhouette. The **electrocardiogram** may be normal. However, cardiac amyloidosis and hemochromatosis are frequently associated with low-voltage QRS complexes. Intraventricular conduction delay and arrhythmias (ventricular and supraventricular) are not uncommon. **Echocardiography** may demonstrate symmetric wall thickening with variable degrees of chamber enlargement. Diffuse hypokinesis may also be noted.

## MANAGEMENT:

The clinical course of patients with restrictive cardiomyopathy usually parallels that of the underlying disease and is generally rapidly progressive and unalterably fatal. The natural history of the idiopathic form is more variable(20). Initial management should be undertaken to alleviate the symptoms of congestive heart failure. It should be noted that cardiac glycosides may precipitate fatal arrhythmias in patients with amyloid heart disease and should be used with caution(21). Additional therapy will be determined by the underlying disease. The cardiac manifestations of hemochromatosis may be improved or alleviated with phlebotomy or chelation therapy. Corticosteroid therapy promotes healing of cardiac sarcoid granulomas but may result in ventricular aneurysm formation. Chemotherapy with alkylating agents is of no proven benefit in patients with cardiac amyloid.

## DIFFERENTIAL DIAGNOSTIC PROBLEMS IN THE ASSESSMENT OF CARDIOMYOPATHIES

A number of other cardiac diseases may present with signs and symptoms similar to those of the cardiomyopathies and thus need to be considered during the course of patient assessment. **Diseases which may "masquerade" as a primary cardiomyopathy include:** rheumatic valvular heart disease, hypertensive heart disease, pericardial effusion, constrictive pericarditis, and coronary artery disease.

**Rheumatic valvular heart disease** should be suspected in the presence of diastolic murmurs which are loudest at the base of the heart or if valvular calcifications are noted on chest x-ray or cardiac fluoroscopy. An apical holosystolic mitral regurgitation murmur which becomes louder after the institution of digoxin or diuretic therapy is suggestive of primary valvular disease.

**Hypertensive heart disease** should be suspected in the presence of a history of systemic arterial hypertension or if there is evidence of other end-organ damage, i.e., retinopathy, renal failure.

**A pericardial effusion with tamponade** may produce symptoms suggestive of congestive heart failure and radiographic evidence of an enlarged cardiac silhouette. Effusion with tamponade should be suspected if a third or fourth heart sound is not audible and low-voltage QRS complexes are noted on the electrocardiogram of a patient with "cardiomegaly." Additional physical findings which should suggest pericardial disease include: pulsus paradoxus, an absent "y" descent of the jugular venous pulse, and distended neck veins without radiographic evidence of pulmonary congestion (see Chapter 14) in a patient with an enlarged cardiac silhouette.

**Constrictive pericarditis** may mimic a restrictive cardiomyopathy. A diagnosis of constrictive pericarditis is favored if pericardial calcifications are noted on chest x-ray and if echocardiography demonstrates normal or nearly normal systolic ventricular function and the absence of chamber enlargement. Constrictive pericarditis is suggested if invasive hemodynamic assessment demonstrates an early diastolic "dip and plateau" configuration of ventricular pressures with equal end-diastolic pressures in both left and right ventricles.

**Coronary artery disease and ischemic heart disease** should be suspected if there is a history of typical angina pectoris or a history of a definite acute myocardial infarction. Coronary artery calcification noted radiographically is likewise suggestive of coronary artery disease. This is the most difficult exclusion, even with currently available noninvasive techniques. It should be recalled that patients with any form of cardiomyopathy, but particularly the hypertrophic type, may relate a history of chest pain which is typical of angina pectoris. In addition, the electrocardiogram of patients with congestive or restrictive forms may demonstrate a "pseudoinfarction" pattern with Q or QS waves. Coronary arteriography should be performed if the diagnosis is not established and specific therapy will be determined by a precise diagnosis.

## REFERENCES

1. Johnson RA, Palacios I: Dilated cardiomyopathies of the adult (Part I). N Engl J Med 307:1051, 1982. Dilated cardiomyopathies of the adult (Part II). N Engl J Med 307:1119, 1982.

2. Fowler NO: Differential diagnosis of cardiomyopathies. Prog Cardiovasc Dis 14:213, 1971.

3. Roberts WC, Perloff JK: Mitral valvular disease. A clinicopathologic survey of the conditions causing the mitral valve to function abnormally. Ann Intern Med 77:939, 1972.

4. Bulkley BH, Roberts WC: Dilatation of the mitral annulus. A rare cause of mitral regurgitation. Am J Med 59:457, 1975.

5. Criley JM, Chambers RD, Blaufuss AH, et al.: Mitral stenosis: Mechanico-acoustical events. In: The Physiologic Principles of Heart Sounds and Murmurs. American Heart Association Monograph, 1974. Dallas, Texas.

6. Criley JM, Siegel RJ: Has "obstruction" hindered our understanding of hypertrophic cardiomyopathy? Circulation 72:1148, 1985.

7. Criley JM, Lennon PA, Abbasi AS, et al.: Hypertrophic cardiomyopathy. In Levine HJ (ed): Clinical Cardiovascular Physiology. New York, Grune and Stratton, Inc., 1976, pp. 771-827.

8. Engler RL, Smith P, LeWinter M, et al.: The electrocardiogram in asymmetric septal hypertrophy. Chest 75:167, 1979.

9. Shah PM: Hypertrophic cardiomyopathy. Ann Rev Med 28:235, 1977.

10. Shah PM, Adelman AG, Wigle ED, et al.: The natural (and unnatural) history of hypertrophic obstructive cardiomyopathy. A multicenter study. Circ Res 34:179, 1974.

11. Frank MJ, Abdulla M, Canedo MI, et al.: Long-term medical management of hypertrophic cardiomyopathy. Am J Cardiol 42:993, 1978.

12. Rosing DR, Condit JR, Maron BJ, et al.: Verapamil therapy: A new approach to the pharmacologic treatment of hypertrophic cardiomyopathy. III. Effects of long-term administration. Am J Cardiol 48:545, 1981.

13. Bonow RO, Dilsizian V, Rosing DR, et al.: Verapamil-induced improvement in left ventricular diastolic filling and increased exercise tolerance in patients with hypertrophic cardiomyopathy: short- and long-term effects. Circulation 72:853, 1985.

14. Epstein SE, Rosing DR: Verapamil: Its potential for causing serious complications in patients with hypertrophic cardiomyopathy. Circulation 64:437, 1981.

15. Benotti JR, Grossman W, Cohn PF: Clinical profile of restrictive cardiomyopathy. Circulation 61:1206, 1980.

16. Meany E, Shabetai R, Bhargava V, et al.: Cardiac amyloidosis, constrictive pericarditis and restrictive cardiomyopathy. Am J Cardiol 38:547, 1976.

17. Siqueira-Filho AG, Cunha CLP, Tajik AJ, et al.: M-mode and two-dimensional echocardiographic features in cardiac amyloidosis. Circulation 63:188, 1981.

18. Nicolosi GL, Pavan D, Lestuzzi C, et al.: Prospective identification of patients with amyloid heart disease by two-dimensional echocardiography. Circulation 70:432, 1984.

19. Roberts, WC, McAllister HA, Ferrans VJ: Sarcoidosis of the heart. Am J Med 63:86, 1977.

20. Siegel RJ, Shah PK, Fishbein MC: Idiopathic restrictive cardiomyopathy. Circulation 70:165, 1984.

21. Rubinow A, Skinner M, Cohen AS: Digoxin sensitivity in amyloid cardiomyopathy. Circulation 63:1285, 1981.

# Chapter 14

# Pericardial
# Heart Disease

The pericardium consists of a serous or loose fibrous membrane (visceral pericardium), beneath which lies the myocardium, and a dense collagenous sac (parietal pericardium) which surrounds the heart. Under normal conditions, up to 50 ml of fluid may be present in the space between the visceral and parietal pericardium. The pericardium supports the heart and limits its movement within the mediastinum, serves as a barrier to the spread of infection from the lungs and pleural space to the myocardium, may limit the degree of atrioventricular valvular insufficiency should sudden cardiac dilatation occur, and may modify the ventricular pressure-volume (compliance) relationship as preload is increased(1,2).

Because its layers are serosal surfaces (lined with mesothelial cells) and due to its proximity and attachments to other structures (pleura, diaphragm, sternum, and myocardium), the pericardium may be involved in a number of systemic or localized disease processes. The clinical presentations of pericardial disease are variable and are dependent not only upon the pericardium's response to an injury (exudation of fluid, fibrin, or inflammatory cells, granuloma formation, fibrous proliferation, or calcification) but also upon how the response affects cardiac function. **The following discussion highlights the clinical presentation and evaluation of acute pericarditis, cardiac tamponade, and constrictive pericarditis.**

## ACUTE PERICARDITIS

**SYMPTOMS AND SIGNS:**

The vast majority of patients with acute pericarditis will complain of retrosternal or precordial **chest pain.** The pain is most often, but not always, **"pleuritic"** in character (worsened with deep inspiration, movement, or lying down), and relieved by sitting up, leaning forward, and by taking shallow inspirations. Since the pain may be aggravated by inspiration, the patient may complain of **shortness of breath.** Additional symptoms most often will be determined by the underlying etiology.

A **pericardial friction rub** is the most common and important physical finding in pericarditis(3). It is **most often triphasic in character**, consisting of a systolic component during ventricular systole, an early diastolic component occurring during the early phase of ventricular filling, and a presystolic component synchronous with atrial systole. **The friction rub is less commonly biphasic**--a systolic component with either an early diastolic or presystolic component. A single component or **monophasic rub is rare** (18% of cases) and is usually systolic. The **friction rub is best heard** at the cardiac apex with the patient sitting up or in the hands-and-knees position. It may be transient and its presence does not preclude a large pericardial effusion.

## CHEST X-RAY (CXR):

A routine chest x-ray may be of value in acute pericarditis, but not necessarily in diagnosis, as heart size may be normal with a small pericardial effusion. The presence of a pericardial friction rub in association with pleuro-pulmonary or mediastinal abnormalities may assist in establishing an etiology, e.g., neoplastic or infectious.

## ELECTROCARDIOGRAM:

The ECG may be diagnostic, especially if followed over time(4). In the **acute phase**(Stage 1), the ST segment vector is directed anteriorly, inferiorly, and leftward, causing **ST segment elevation** (reflecting subepicardial injury) in the precordial leads, especially in V5 and V6 and in leads I and II (Chapter 1, Figure 1.4). ST segment elevation in V6 is usually greater than 25% of the T wave amplitude(5). An isoelectric or depressed ST segment is commonly seen in V1. PR segment depression may be noted in leads II, aVF, and V4-V6. In **Stage 2** the ST segment begins returning to the isoelectric line and T wave amplitude decreases. **T wave inversion** in those leads previously showing ST segment elevation is noted during **Stage 3**. At this time the ST segment is isoelectric. **Stage 4** is characterized by resolution of the electrocardiographic abnormalities. Additional ECG abnormalities may be noted during pericarditis and include **atrial arrhythmias** (usually insignificant)(6) and, if a large effusion is present, **low-voltage QRS complexes** and **electrical alternans**(7). The latter phenomena are due to the "insulating" effect of the pericardial fluid and the pendulum motion of the heart within the pericardium at a frequency one-half of the heart rate.

Common causes of pericarditis/pericardial effusion include(8):

1. **Idiopathic**. Commonly preceded by a febrile illness or "viral syndrome." In most cases, the etiology is not established.

2. **Infections**. **Viral**--Coxsackie (especially group B), echo virus, influenza,and the herpes viruses. Frequently viral pericarditis is associated with a myocarditis and cardiac enzyme elevation; in this instance, the term myopericarditis is used. **Bacterial**--usually the result of spread from a contiguous myocardial abscess or

pleuropulmonary focus or after thoracic surgery or trauma. **Staphylococcus aureus** and **streptococcus pneumoniae** are the most common organisms. Tuberculosis used to be a common etiology of pericarditis, but is now relatively rare. Pericarditis may occur during acute rheumatic fever. **Fungal--Histoplasma capsulatum.**

3. **Connective Tissue Disease.** Rheumatoid arthritis, systemic lupus, scleroderma, polyarteritis.

4. **Malignancy.** Most commonly metastatic from breast or lung. However, lymphoma, leukemia, and melanoma have a high incidence of metastasis to the pericardium.

5. **Uremia.** Usually treatable by dialysis or more frequent dialysis in those already on dialysis.

6. **Drug-Induced.** "Lupus syndrome" due to procainamide, hydralazine, isoniazid, or diphenylhydantoin. The anthracycline antineoplastic agents, such as doxorubicin, may cause pericarditis in addition to the more common myocardial toxicity.

7. **Post-Myocardial Infarction (Dressler's Syndrome).** Syndrome of fever, pericarditis, and pleuritis that occurs weeks to months after a myocardial infarction. This may have an immunologic basis and is different than the acute pericarditis that can occur within the first week after a transmural myocardial infarction.

8. **Post-Pericardiotomy.** Incidence as high as 30% within 2 to 4 weeks after open heart surgery, often associated with pulmonary infiltrate and/or pleural effusion.

9. **Mediastinal Radiation Therapy.**

10. **Myxedema.**

11. **Sarcoidosis.**

**LABORATORY ASSESSMENT:**

In addition to careful history and physical examination, the following laboratory studies may be of value in establishing an etiologic diagnosis.

1. Complete blood count (CBC) and differential: May suggest infection or leukemia.

2. Erythrocyte sedimentation rate (ESR): Usually elevated, may be useful in following course and assessing response to therapy.

3. Blood urea nitrogen/creatinine.

4.  Electrocardiogram.

5.  Streptococcal serology.

6.  Blood cultures.

7.  Serology: Acute and convalescent viral titers, antinuclear antibody (ANA), double-stranded DNA, RA latex, hepatitis B surface antigen (frequently positive in patients with polyarteritis nodosum).

8.  TB skin test.

9.  Echocardiography:  To confirm the presence of pericardial fluid and rule out a contiguous cardiac process (endocarditis, myocardial abscess).

10. Pericardiocentesis:  Indicated in suspected cardiac tamponade and occasionally indicated as a diagnostic procedure, especially if infection or malignancy is suspected.

**THERAPY:**

Therapy is most appropriately directed at the underlying etiology if a treatable cause can be defined.   Chest pain may be alleviated with the use of salicylates or nonsteroidal anti-inflammatory drugs. Corticosteroid therapy for several days may be necessary to treat severe pain.    Patients with viral myopericarditis should be placed at bed rest and frequently assessed for signs and symptoms of declining left ventricular function.  Echocardiography may be helpful in differentiating depressed myocardial contractility from cardiac tamponade or constriction.  Corticosteroids have been instilled directly into the pericardial space to treat uremic pericarditis.  Instillation of antineoplastic agents or sclerosing agents into the pericardial space has been used in malignant causes of pericarditis.

It is not unusual for the patient to have one or more relapses of acute symptoms weeks or months after apparent resolution.  If these episodes continue to recur, a trial of corticosteroid therapy may be more effective than other anti-inflammatory drugs.  Rarely, pericardiectomy is indicated to relieve recurrent symptoms or as prophylaxis against constrictive pericarditis.

## CARDIAC TAMPONADE

Intrapericardial pressure is normally subatmospheric.  An increase in the quantity of intrapericardial fluid, whatever the cause, results in a rise in the intrapericardial pressure.  The initial portion of the pericardial pressure-volume curve is relatively flat(2); i.e., relatively large increases in intrapericardial volume produce small changes in intrapericardial pressure.  The curve becomes steeper as the fibrous and relatively inelastic parietal pericardium is "stretched." Eventually, continued fluid accumulation will raise the intrapericardial pressure to a level which exceeds the normal filling pressure of the ventricles. When this occurs, ventricular filling is restricted and "cardiac tamponade" is present. The slope of the pericardial pressure-volume curve and the point at which cardiac tamponade occurs is dependent upon:

1. **The Rate of Fluid Accumulation.** With slow accumulation, large volumes of fluid can be more readily accommodated due to gradual stretching of the pericardium.

2. **Pericardial Compliance.** A previously diseased and thickened pericardium is likely to be less distensible.

3. **Intravascular Volume.** Tamponade will inhibit cardiac output to a greater extent during hypovolemia.

The pathophysiology of cardiac tamponade is complex, yet explains a number of physical and hemodynamic findings. Pulsus paradoxus is one of the most consistent and important clinical features of cardiac tamponade. An understanding of its genesis may be of help in understanding the physiology of tamponade.

**PULSUS PARADOXUS:**

As originally described in constrictive pericarditis, a paradoxical arterial pulse is said to be present when the cardiac rhythm is regular and there are apparent "dropped beats" in the peripheral pulse during inspiration. Manometrically, pulsus paradoxus is present when there is a greater than 10 mm Hg decrease in systolic blood pressure during inspiration in the supine position. A few mm Hg of inspiratory decrease in arterial pressure is normal(9).

Pulsus paradoxus results from the inspiratory decrease in left ventricular filling, caused by the dominance of augmented right heart filling (during inspiration) in the confined intrapericardial space. Inspiration creates a negative intrathoracic pressure that causes the left heart filling pressure to fall. As the pulmonary vasculature becomes more compliant and the left atrium and its tributaries are subjected to a negative pressure, the overfilled extrathoracic systemic venous reservoir provides a more constant pressure head for right heart filling. Thus, the right heart dominates the limited intrapericardial cardiovascular space during inspiration and this augmented filling is translated into increased right heart output, which in turn causes a rise in left heart filling pressure as inspiration ends and expiration begins(10).

Figure 14.1 demonstrates the phasic swings in left heart filling pressure (pulmonary capillary wedge [PCW]) and the relatively constant right atrial pressure (RA), resulting in inspiratory inhibition of left heart filling and marked decrease in arterial pulse amplitude--the paradoxical pulse. During apnea, there is an equilibration of atrial pressures, with "equal sharing" of the limited intrapericardial space and a steady arterial pressure.

**Figure 14.1**

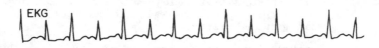

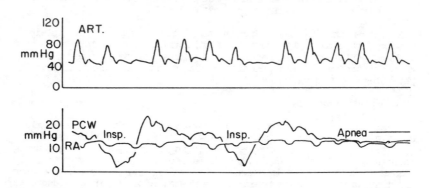

From the description of the mechanism of pulsus paradoxus, it should be apparent that ventricular filling in tamponade and constrictive pericarditis is dependent upon systemic venous pressure(11).

**Pulsus paradoxus is not diagnostic of cardiac tamponade and it may be noted in constrictive pericarditis, restrictive cardiomyopathy, shock, pulmonary embolism, asthma, or severe obstructive airway disease and tension pneumothorax.** It may be absent in tamponade if the patient is hypovolemic (low pressure tamponade)(12), with tamponade complicating chronic left ventricular dysfunction manifested by elevated left ventricular (LV) diastolic pressure(13) (see below) or if the patient has an atrial septal defect(14).

## IMPORTANT CLINICAL FEATURES IN CARDIAC TAMPONADE:

The symptoms associated with cardiac tamponade are nonspecific. The patient will most commonly complain of intolerance to minimal activity and dyspnea. Congestive failure might well be diagnosed and inappropriate and potentially dangerous therapy (diuresis) instituted if a careful history and attention to salient physical findings are ignored. **Cardiac tamponade should be suspected in the hemodynamically compromised patient:**

-   With known pericarditis.

-   Following blunt or penetrating chest trauma.

-   Following open-heart surgery or cardiac catheterization.

-   With known or suspected intrathoracic neoplasm.

-   With a suspected dissecting aortic aneurysm.

**Physical examination** commonly reveals a decreased systolic blood pressure with a narrow pulse pressure and pulsus paradoxus. The neck veins are distended, and examination of jugular venous pulsations reveals a rapid "x" descent and attenuated or absent "y" descent. Tachycardia, a compensatory mechanism to maintain cardiac output, is usually present. The apical impulse is indistinct and the lateral border of cardiac dullness is displaced laterally. Cardiac auscultation commonly demonstrates "distant" heart sounds. Pulmonary rales are uncommon, but a pleural effusion may be present. There may be right upper quadrant tenderness due to hepatic engorgement.

**Chest x-ray** may or may not demonstrate enlargement of the cardiac shadow, depending upon the volume of intrapericardial fluid. The rapid accumulation of a relatively small amount of pericardial fluid may produce tamponade with minimal enlargement of the cardiac silhouette. On the lateral chest x-ray, an epicardial fat pad line may be seen within the cardiac silhouette. The pulmonary vasculature usually appears normal. Additional chest x-ray findings will be dependent upon the etiology, such as mediastinal adenopathy, a lung mass or infiltrate, etc.

The **electrocardiogram** may demonstrate low-voltage QRS complexes, ST segment elevation, and PR segment depression characteristic of pericarditis or electrical alternans (beat-to-beat variation in P, R, and T wave amplitude). Alternans is seen in only 10-20% of cases of tamponade and 50-60% of these cases are neoplastic in origin[15].

**Echocardiography** demonstrates intrapericardial fluid. The heart may appear to "swing" within the pericardial space if there is a large amount of pericardial fluid. Obliteration of the right ventricular cavity may be seen as the anterior wall of the right ventricle and the intraventricular septum approximate one another in systole[16-19]. Right atrial compression by intrapericardial fluid has also been described[20,21].

If **cardiac catheterization** is performed, equalization of right atrial, right ventricular, pulmonary artery diastolic, pulmonary capillary wedge or left atrial, and left ventricular end-diastolic pressures will be recorded during suspended respiration (Figure 14.1). The intracardiac diastolic pressure will approximate intrapericardial pressure. A "dip and plateau" configuration of ventricular pressure, characteristic of constrictive pericarditis and restrictive cardiomyopathy, is not seen.

Recent studies indicate that in some patients with clinical tamponade, pulsus paradoxus, and equalization of intracardiac diastolic pressures may be absent(13). This is most likely to occur in patients with intrinsically elevated LV diastolic pressure as might occur with chronic hypertension. Pulsus paradoxus is not found because resistance to LV filling is constant throughout the respiratory cycle and equalization of diastolic pressures is noted only in the right heart chambers, with LV pressure being higher than right heart pressures. Thus, the absence of pulsus paradoxus and classic hemodynamic findings does not rule out tamponade.

## ETIOLOGY:

Cardiac tamponade may occur during the course of acute pericarditis of any cause but is most commonly encountered following chest trauma, cardiac surgery, and with neoplastic involvement of the pericardium(22).

## TREATMENT:

Volume expansion with normal saline will usually increase cardiac output and blood pressure but is, at best, only a temporary measure. Pericardiocentesis may dramatically improve the hemodynamic status of the compromised patient.

**Pericardiocentesis** is a lifesaving procedure in patients with tamponade, but the procedure is potentially hazardous and should be performed with considerable care and under optimal circumstances. The potential hazards of cardiac perforation and coronary artery laceration can be minimized, and the therapeutic and diagnostic yield can be enhanced by appropriate planning and attention to detail.

Pericardiocentesis should be performed in the cardiac catheterization laboratory whenever circumstances permit. The availability of fluoroscopy, a defibrillator, adequate laboratory facilities (e.g., hematocrit centrifuge), and the ease of ECG and pressure monitoring and recording in such a setting enhance the safety and diagnostic yield.

Whenever possible, pressure from a pulmonary artery or right atrial catheter should be monitored before, during, and after pericardiocentesis. The presence of tamponade may be confirmed by a prompt decrease in central venous pressure attendant with pericardial fluid aspiration and the recurrence of tamponade can be detected by an elevation of right heart pressures toward pre-pericardiocentesis levels.

The patient's anterior chest wall and epigastrium are prepared with an iodine prep and a large sterile drape is applied.  The limb leads of a three-channel ECG patient cable are attached to the extremities and precordial electrodes are placed in the V5 and V6 positions (lateral to the sterile drape).  After infiltration with local anesthesia in the subxiphoid area, a long, plastic-sheathed, 18 gauge needle is attached to a lidocaine-filled syringe via a metal three-way stopcock.  One end of a sterile alligator clip is placed on the stopcock or needle and the other end on the V4 electrode cable, preferably using a self-grounding three-wire lead.

As the metal needle tip is placed in the subcutaneous tissue beneath the xiphoid process, the "V4-5-6" lead selector of the ECG machine should be turned on and a continuous recording made to ascertain that a reliable complex can be obtained from the"V4" exploring needle electrode.  The needle is then advanced toward the right scapula, infiltrating with lidocaine (for anesthesia and to keep the needle patent), stopping after every few millimeters to monitor the exploring ECG lead and to aspirate for pericardial fluid.

If the needle touches atrial tissue, there will be a large P wave complex and elevation of the P-R segment.  If the ventriclar myocardium is encountered, the QRS complex will be large and the ST segment will be elevated.  The simultaneous recording of surface leads (V5 and V6) will aid in identifying the complexes recorded from the exploring electrode. If myocardium is encountered with the needle, it should be withdrawn during gentle aspiration.

If pericardial fluid is encountered, a 30-ml syringe can be attached to the sidearm of the three-way stopcock and a sample withdrawn.  The beneficial effect of pericardial fluid withdrawal on venous pressure or on the magnitude of pulsus paradoxus is often seen upon withdrawal of less than 100 ml of fluid.  If fluid is easily withdrawn, a plastic sheath may be advanced over the needle, minimizing the hazard of further pericardiocentesis but negating further monitoring of the exploring ECG lead.  **The aspirated fluid should be examined carefully and immediately placed in sterile tubes for laboratory analysis** (bacterial, fungal, and mycobacterial cultures, protein content, cytology, cell count, hematocrit).  **If the fluid is grossly bloody, an immediate hematocrit should be performed concurrently with a blood sample to make certain that the fluid being withdrawn is not from an intracardiac source.** A rapid assessment can be made by expelling a small quantity of fluid on a gauze sponge.  If it has the color, clarity, and consistency of red wine, it is most probably hemolyzed blood from the pericardial space.  On the other hand, if it is thick and rapidly forms a clot, it may be blood from a vascular compartment. **Up to 70% of malignant pericardial effusions can be diagnosed by fluid cytology.**

It is often useful to inject 5-10 ml of radiographic contrast medium into the pericardial space. This will opacify the fluid and permit an estimate of the adequacy of the pericardiocentesis during fluoroscopy.

If rapid fluid reaccumulation is anticipated (as in a suspected metastatic malignancy), it is helpful to insert a guide-wire through the plastic needle sheath while there is free fluid in the pericardial space. A "pig-tail" catheter with multiple side holes can be inserted over the guide wire into the pericardial space. This catheter is less likely to become occluded than the plastic sheath and can be left in place for several days for repeated fluid withdrawals or medication instillation. The catheter should be removed if there is evidence of cardiac rhythm disturbance, notably frequent premature beats or atrial fibrillation.

As noted above, if there is tamponade, monitoring of right heart pressures will confirm the diagnosis since withdrawal of fluid will cause a prompt fall in filling pressure. If there is no fall in venous pressure despite fluid removal, the diagnosis of tamponade is in doubt.

## CONSTRICTIVE PERICARDITIS

**Constrictive pericarditis is clinically and pathologically distinct from acute pericarditis.** Following pericardial injury, a chronic reparative process characterized by fibrous thickening of the layers of the pericardium may occur. When this process advances to the point where diastolic filling of the normally distensible cardiac chambers is prevented by a nondistensible, thickened pericardium, "constriction" is said to be present. By its nature, constrictive pericarditis is most commonly a chronic process and the end result of a remote and/or occult episode of acute pericarditis. However, clinical manifestations may occur early if fluid accumulates between the thickened layers of pericardium ("effusive, constrictive pericarditis")(23). Constriction may occur following any acute pericardial injury but is more commonly seen following cardiac trauma with intrapericardial hemorrhage, pericardi-otomy (heart surgery), fungal or tuberculous pericarditis, or with uremia. **In the majority of cases, a specific etiology is never determined.**

### SIGNS AND SYMPTOMS:

The patient with constrictive pericarditis most commonly presents with symptoms which mimic congestive heart failure; edema and ascites are often more pronounced than orthopnea and dyspnea. **Careful physical examination** may provide the initial clues to the presence of constrictive pericarditis.  **Pulsus paradoxus** may or may not be present. Although the neck veins are distended, the lungs are clear, the heart is not enlarged, and the precordium is not overactive.  Examination of the jugular venous pulsations reveals a **rapid "y" descent.  Kussmaul's sign**, inspiratory increase in venous pressure, may be noted.  On cardiac auscultation, an early diastolic sound, a **pericardial knock** 60 to 120 msec after the second heart sound may be heard.  A pericardial knock occurs later than an opening snap and slightly earlier than an S3 which it may mimic.  Hepatosplenomegaly may be present along with ascites.

The **chest x-ray** most commonly shows a normal or slightly enlarged cardiac silhouette and clear lung fields with normal pulmonary vasculature.  Pericardial calcification may be seen in approximately 50% of patients with constrictive pericarditis and is best seen on a lateral chest x-ray.

The **electrocardiogram** shows no diagnostic features.

**Echocardiography** occasionally demonstrates pericardial thickening(24).  Septal motion may be abnormal and the left ventricular wall shows abrupt cessation of outward motion during early diastole.

**Cardiac catheterization and hemodynamic assessment is the most important diagnostic study.  Typical hemodynamic features include(25):**

1.  Rapid "x" and "y" descent in the right atrial pressure trace.

2.  Early diastolic pressure "dip and plateau" configuration in the right ventricle (Figure 14.2).

3.  Equalization of increased diastolic pressures in the right atrium, right ventricle, LV, and  pulmonary artery.

4.  Elevated right ventricular and pulmonary arterial pressures.

Figure 14.2

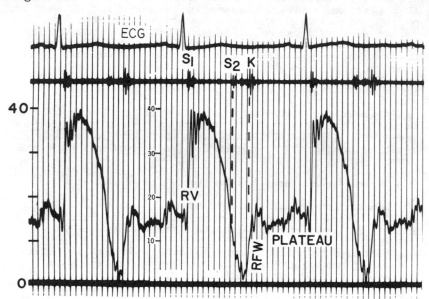

The characteristic diastole "dip and plateau" or "square wave" configuration of right ventricular (RV) pressure in constrictive pericarditis is demonstrated. A similar configuration was noted in the left ventricle. At the onset of diastole, inflow into the ventricles from the distended atria is rapid, producing an abrupt increase in intraventricular pressure corresponding to the rapid filling wave (RFW) shown in the figure. Later diastolic inflow is inhibited as the expanding ventricles encounter noncompliant pericardium. Early equalization of atrial and ventricular pressures and the near cessation of diastolic inflow result in a high-pressure plateau of equal magnitude in all cardiac chambers. A simultaneous phonocardiogram demonstrates the presence of a diastolic knock (K) occurring approximately 0.12 sec after the second heart sound (S2). This sound is heard during the rapid-filling phase of diastole as ventricular filling is suddenly inhibited by the constricting pericardium (time lines = 0.04 sec).

These hemodynamic findings are by no means diagnostic of constrictive pericarditis. Similar pressures may be noted in patients with restrictive cardiomyopathy. Left heart catheterization may serve to differentiate between the two (see Chapter 13, The Cardiomyopathies).

**THERAPY:**

Surgical pericardial stripping is generally effective in symptomatic individuals.

## REFERENCES

1. Shabetai R: The pericardium: An essay on some recent developments. Am J Cardiol 42:1036, 1978.

2. Boltwood CM, Shah PM: The pericardium in health and disease. Curr Prob Cardiol 9:9, 1984.

3. Spodick DH: Pericardial friction rub-characteristics of pericardial rubs in 50 consecutive, prospectively studied patients. N Engl J Med 278:1204, 1968.

4. Suravicz B, Lasseter KC: Electrocardiogram in pericarditis. Am J Cardiol 26:471, 1970.

5. Ginzton LE, Laks MM: The differential diagnosis of acute pericarditis from the normal variant: New electrocardiographic criteria. Circulation 65:1004, 1982.

6. Spodick DH: Frequency of arrhythmias in acute pericarditis determined by Holter monitoring. Am J Cardiol 53:842, 1984.

7. Berger M, Bobak L, Jelveh M, et al.: Pericardial effusion diagnosed by echocardiography. Clinical and electrocardiographic findings in 171 patients. Chest 74:174, 1978.

8. Roberts WC, Spray TL: Pericardial heart disease. Curr Prob Cardiol 2:6, 1977.

9. Reeve R, Reeve FJS, Lin TK: Paradoxical pulse-revisited. Am Heart J 92:120, 1976.

10. McGregor M: Pulsus paradoxus. N Engl J Med 301:480, 1979.

11. Cogswell TL, Bernath GA, Wann S, et al.: Effects of intravascular volume state on the value of pulsus paradoxus and right ventricular diastolic collapse in predicting cardiac tamponade. Circulation 72:1076, 1985.

12. Antman EM, Cargill V, Grossman W: Low-pressure cardiac tamponade. Ann Intern Med 91:403, 1979.

13. Reddy PS, Curtiss EI, O'Toole JD, et al.: Cardiac tamponade: Hemodynamic observations in man. Circulation 58:265, 1978.

14. Winer HE, Kronzon I: Absence of paradoxical pulse in patients with cardiac tamponade and atrial septal defects. Am J Cardiol 44:378, 1979.

15. Theologides A: Neoplastic cardiac tamponade. Semin Oncol 5:181, 1978.

16. Schiller NB, Botuinick EH: Right ventricular compression as a sign of cardiac tamponade. Circulation 56:774, 1977.

17. Settle HP, Adolph RJ, Folwer NO, et al.: Echocardiographic study of cardiac tamponade. Circulation 56:951, 1977.

18. Gaffney FA, Keller AM, Peshock RM, et al.: Pathophysiologic mechanisms of cardiac tamponade and pulsus alternans shown by echocardiography. Am J Cardiol 53:1662, 1984.

19. Kloppenstein HS, Schuchard GH, Wann LS, et al.: The relative merits of pulsus paradoxus and right ventricular diastolic collapse in the early detection of cardiac tamponade: An experimental echocardiographic study. Circulation 71:829, 1985.

20. Singh S, Wann LS, Schuchard GH, et al.: Right ventricular and right atrial collapse in patients with cardiac tamponade--a combined echocardiographic and hemodynamic study. Circulation 70:966, 1984.

21. Fowler NO, Gabel M: The hemodynamic effects of cardiac tamponade: Mainly the result of atrial, not ventricular, compression. Circulation 71:154, 1985.

22. Guberman BA, Fowler NO, Engel PJ, et al.: Cardiac tamponade in medical patients. Circulation 64:633, 1981.

23. Hancock EW: Subacute effusive-constrictive pericarditis. Circulation 43:183, 1971.

24. Voelkel AG, Pietro DA, Polland ED, et al.: Echocardiographic features of constrictive pericarditis. Circulation 58:871 1978.

25. Shabetai R, Fowler NO, Guntheroth WG: The hemodynamics of cardiac tamponade and constrictive pericarditis. Am J Cardiol 16:480, 1970.

# Chapter 15

# Sudden Cardiac Death

## DEFINITION

There is no universally accepted definition of sudden cardiac death. Most investigators define sudden death as an unexpected, nontraumatic non-self-inflicted fatality occurring within 24 hours of the onset of acute symptoms(1). Others have a more strict definition: death occurring within 1 hour of the onset of symptoms(2).

## SCOPE OF THE PROBLEM

Semantic problems regarding definition notwithstanding, sudden cardiac death is the leading cause of death in the United States, claiming approximately 400,000 victims annually, 1,100 lives daily, or almost 1 victim every minute! Approximately 25% of victims have had no prior symptoms of heart disease, and sudden death is often the first indication of clinical heart disease(3).

## ETIOLOGY

Authorities agree that coronary artery disease (CAD) is by far the most common cause of sudden death. When sudden death is defined as death within 24 hours of the onset of symptoms, approximately 60% of cases can be ascribed to CAD(4). When defined as death occurring within an hour of the onset of symptoms, 91% of cases can be attributed to CAD(5). Sudden death should not be equated with "a massive heart attack" since the majority of victims have not suffered a myocardial infarction(5,6).

Table 15.1
Typical Characteristics of Sudden Death Syndrome

Sex . . . . . . . . . . . . . . . . . Male (median age, 59)

Place of occurrence . . . . . . . . Outside of hospital

Prodrome. . . . . . . . . . . . . . Absent
                                    75% during non-
                                    strenuous activity

                                    25% during or after
                                    vigorous activity

Acute coronary occlusion. . . . . . Absent

Severe CAD. . . . . . . . . . . . . Present

Left ventricular dysfunction. . . . . Present

Chronic ventricular ectopy. . . . . Present

Recurrence of ventricular
      fibrillation . . . . . . . . . . *Up to 30% (1 year
                                        follow-up)

*Highest in resuscitated victims of sudden death who have
not had an acute transmural myocardial infarction.


Other less common disease entities which may culminate in sudden
cardiac death include:

1. **Congenital:**

   - Prolonged QT syndromes (Romano-Ward syndrome, if autosomal
   dominant without deafness; Jervell and Lange-Nielsen syndrome if
   autosomal recessive with congenital deafness).

   - Congenital heart disease:  Hypertrophic cardiomyopathy, aortic
   stenosis, anomalies of the coronary circulation, Ebstein's
   anomaly, mitral valve prolapse.

   - Conduction abnormalities:  Preexcitation syndromes, such as
   Wolff-Parkinson-White syndrome; heart block.

2. **Acquired (in addition to CAD):**

   - Aortic stenosis.

   - Prinzmetal's angina.

   - Conduction abnormalities (Lev's or Lenegre's disease).

- Iatrogenic misadventures: digoxin toxicity, kaluretic diuretics, antiarrhythmic drug toxicity ("quinidine syncope"), liquid protein diets, tricyclic antidepressants and phenothiazines, inappropriate pacemaker implants, or malfunction of permanent pacemakers.

- Aortic dissection.

- Pulmonary embolism.

- Coronary artery embolism.

## PATHOPHYSIOLOGY OF SUDDEN CARDIAC DEATH

Although severe CAD (>70% occlusion of one or more of the three major epicardial vessels) is found in the majority of victims of sudden death, only a minority (15-33%) will have pathologic evidence of an acute coronary occlusion or recent myocardial infarction(5-7). **The fact that an acute coronary occlusion is found in only a minority of cases suggests that a "functional" rather than a "mechanical" (anatomic) abnormality is the underlying problem.** Arrhythmia monitoring and detection during in-hospital and out-of-hospital resuscitation of the sudden death victim has provided evidence that primary ventricular fibrillation is the electrophysiologic event which most often precipitates sudden death. Ventricular fibrillation frequently occurs on a background of chronic electrical instability which may manifest itself as premature ventricular contractions (PVCs). If PVCs are truly harbingers of sudden death, antiarrhythmic drug therapy and suppression of PVCs should decrease the incidence of sudden death in the population at risk. Although limited to selected subpopulations, there is some clinical data to support this "PVC hypothesis"(8-11).

## LIMITATIONS OF THE PVC HYPOTHESIS

Clinical studies indicate that there is considerable spontaneous variation in the frequency and complexity of PVCs during ambulatory electrocardiographic monitoring(12). PVCs thus appear to be an unstable variable and this spontaneous variation complicates the evaluation of antiarrhythmic drug response and assessment of efficacy in clinical trials. Detailed analysis of sequential 24-hour ECG recordings during control periods and during antiarrhythmic drug therapy suggests that an 83% reduction in PVCs needs to be demonstrated before one can state that a drug is causing the reduction(12).

**It is uncertain to what extent PVCs must be suppressed to protect against sudden death.** It may be possible to prevent the recurrence of advanced ventricular arrhythmias and sudden death with drug therapy without suppressing all PVCs(13).

There may be little correlation (2%) between symptoms and advanced grades of PVCs occurring during 24-hour ambulatory monitoring(14). Therefore, aggressive treatment of PVCs in a patient with symptoms (i.e., syncope) may not alleviate the symptoms.

**An electrophysiologically unstable myocardium appears to be a required substrate for ventricular fibrillation and sudden death.** PVCs in this setting may be either a catalyst for repetitive activity and fibrillation or a benign marker of electrical instability. Antiarrhythmic drug therapy and suppression of PVCs would be beneficial only if PVCs are the trigger for the ultimate electrical catastrophe. A more direct and clinically applicable means of detecting the electrophysiologic abnormality which places the myocardium at risk for fibrillation is needed.

## APPROACHES TO THE PROBLEM OF SUDDEN DEATH

Current research dealing with the problem of sudden death has been directed toward identifying the population at risk and determining the effect of pharmacologic interventions on recurrence and longevity(15).

### THE SUBJECT AT RISK:

Premature ventricular contractions are ubiquitous and occur even in the absence of overt heart disease. The method used to detect PVCs will determine their frequency in a given population. If a standard 12-lead electrocardiogram is used, 0.8% of healthy individuals will have PVCs(16). If 24-hour ambulatory monitoring (Holter monitoring) is used, 50% of healthy individuals will have PVCs, although the PVCs are usually few in number and rarely multiform in configuration(17). The mere presence or absence of PVCs is not by itself predictive of future sudden cardiac death. Thus, **detection of PVCs does not necessarily mandate pharmacologic intervention. PVCs should only be treated if they are symptomatic or if they are felt to place the patient at risk for sudden cardiac death,** such as following a myocardial infarction or in the presence of organic heart disease, and in survivors of cardiac arrest(15).

Most authorities agree that the occurrence of sudden death in the population at greatest risk, i.e., those with underlying heart disease, is related to the frequency or complexity of ventricular arrhythmias. A number of "grading" systems have been proposed. Implicit to all grading systems is the belief that "high" grades of PVCs enhance the risk of future sudden death. The **grading system of Lown**(18), or a modification of it, is the most frequently used:

| Grade | Characteristics |
|-------|-----------------|
| 0 | No PVCs |
| 1A | Occasional, isolated PVCs (less than 30/hr, less than 1/min) |
| 1B | Occasional isolated PVCs (less than 30/hr, more than 1/min) |
| 2 | Frequent PVCs (more than 30/hr) |
| 3 | Multiform PVCs |
| 4A | Repetitive PVCs; couplets |
| 4B | Repetitive PVCs; salvos of 3 or more in a row |
| 5 | Early PVCs (i.e., abutting or interrupting the T wave) |

It has been shown that the presence of complex ventricular ectopy (Grades 3-5) in survivors of myocardial infarction is associated with a two or three-fold increase in the incidence rate of sudden death during a 3-year follow-up period(19).

The routine risk factors for CAD do not define a special subpopulation prone to sudden death. Among patients with CAD, left ventricular dysfunction (depressed ejection fraction) and ventricular arrhythmias are probably interrelated risk factors for sudden death(20,21).

**TREATMENT:**

At present it is uncertain if drug control of advanced or high grades of PVCs decreases the incidence of sudden cardiac death in all patients in whom they are demonstrated. **Treatment is not indicated in asymptomatic, healthy individuals**(22). There is no substantial evidence to support the contention that antiarrhythmic drugs increase longevity of patients with chronic CAD and asymptomatic PVCs. Since there is no readily available means to identify the patient at high risk for sudden death, **it would seem prudent, based on present limited information, to initiate long-term antiarrhythmic drug therapy in the following subgroups of patients with PVCs**(3,15):

1. Patients who develop ventricular fibrillation which is not the direct result of an acute myocardial infarction. This is the highest risk group with a 30-35% risk of sudden death within 12 months, if untreated.

2. Patients with known CAD (with or without congestive heart failure) and ventricular tachycardia of more than 3 beats during ambulatory ECG monitoring or exercise testing.

3. Patients who have sustained a myocardial infarction during the preceding 12 months and in whom Grades 3-5 PVCs are demonstrated.

4. Patients with Grades 3-5 PVCs and greater than or equal to 2-mm ST segment depression or chest pain on exercise stress testing or monitoring.

5. Patients with a prolonged QT syndrome with greater than or equal to Grade 2 PVCs if associated with syncope or presyncope and if there is a family history of sudden death.

6. Symptomatic patients with mitral valve prolapse and Grades 3-5 PVCs, especially if there is a history of syncope.

7. Patients with hypertrophic cardiomyopathy with Grades 3-5 PVCs, syncope, or a family history of sudden death.

8. Patients with PVCs and disabling symptoms in the absence of overt heart disease.

## MANAGEMENT OF SUDDEN DEATH SURVIVORS

In patients who have been resuscitated from ventricular fibrillation or who have recurrent bouts of hemodynamically significant ventricular tachycardia, a more **aggressive management program** should be pursued(15).

In those patients who have frequent and advanced grades of ventricular ectopy on monitoring, **noninvasive, acute drug testing protocols** can be used(23). Acute oral loading of an antiarrhythmic drug is employed along with exercise testing and 24-hour monitoring. The goal of therapy is to suppress all Grades 4 and 5 PVCs and to reduce ventricular couplets to 10% of their original frequency. Occasionally, drugs such as quinidine or procainamide may actually worsen the rhythm ("pro-arrhythmic effect").

In those patients who do not have frequent high-grade ventricular ectopy on monitoring, **programmed electrical stimulation** of the heart can be performed. This consists of invasive testing with one to three extra stimuli added after ventricular pacing at various ventricular sites to provoke sustained ventricular tachycardia (VT). In those patients who develop VT with stimulation, the efficacy of an antiarrhythmic drug is judged by its ability to prevent sustained VT during repeat stimulation(24). Both the noninvasive and invasive methods have been shown to reduce mortality, if an acceptable antiarrhythmic drug is found.

Various **surgical techniques** have been employed to treat high-grade ventricular ectopy unresponsive to oral antiarrhythmics. Coronary artery bypass surgery effectively treats some patients who presumably have an ischemic origin to the ectopy.  This can also be combined with an aneurysmectomy, if needed, since the edges of aneurysms may be foci for re-entry.  Endocardial mapping techniques can localize the anatomical site of origin of ectopic foci more precisely to allow endocardial resection of a localized area(25).

**Pacemakers** have been used that pace using extra stimuli or burst pacing to terminate ventricular tachycardia.  Recently, automatic implantable defibrillators have been developed that can recognize and internally defibrillate ventricular fibrillation soon after its initiation (see Chapter 17, Artificial Cardiac Pacemakers).

## PREDICTING SUDDEN DEATH AFTER MYOCARDIAL INFARCTION

Sudden cardiac death accounts for >50% of cardiac mortality following MI.  Several large clinical studies have identified **"risk factors" associated with an increased prevalence of post-MI sudden death**(26,27):  1) severe left ventricular dysfunction, 2) significant multivessel coronary artery disease, 3) high-grade ventricular ectopy, 4) the ability to initiate sustained ventricular tachycardia with programmed electrical stimulation, and 5) the presence of two separate areas of infarction.  Indications for electrophysiologic testing after MI are presently controversial.

**Several large studies using various beta blockers** (propranolol, timolol, and metoprolol) **have shown that treatment with these agents within 1 to 6 weeks after a myocardial infarction can significantly reduce one year mortality**(28-30).  The mechanism is a reduction in the incidence of sudden death which may be due to an increase in the ventricular fibrillation threshold or antiarrhythmic effects of the beta blockers.

### REFERENCES

1.  Paul O, Schatz M:  On sudden death.  Circulation 43:7,1971.

2.  Goldstein S:  The necessity of a uniform definition of sudden coronary death:  Witnessed death within 1 hour of the onset of acute symptoms.  Am Heart J 103:156, 1982.

3.  Lown B:  Sudden cardiac death:  The major challenge confronting contemporary cardiology. Am J Cardiol 43:313, 1979.

4.  Kuller L, Lilienfield A, Fisher R:  Epidemiologic study of sudden and unexpected death due to arteriosclerotic heart disease. Circulation 34:1056, 1966.

5.  Reichenbach D, Moss N, Meyer E:  Pathology of the heart in sudden cardiac death.  Am J Cardiol 39:865, 1977.

6.  Schwartz CJ, Gerrity RG:  Anatomic pathology of sudden unexpected cardiac death.  Circulation 52:III-18, 1975.

7.  Cobb LA, Werner JA, Trobough GB:  Sudden cardiac death.  I.  A decade's experience with out-of-hospital resuscitation.  Modern Concepts Cardiovasc Dis 49:31, 1980.

8.  Myerburg RJ, Condi C, Sheps DS, et al.:  Antiarrhythmic drug therapy in survivors of prehospital cardiac arrest:  Comparison of effects on chronic ventricular arrhythmias and on recurrent cardiac arrest. Circulation 59:855, 1979.

9.  Ruskin JN, DiMarco JP, Garan H:  Out-of-hospital cardiac arrest. Electrophysiologic observations and selection of long-term antiarrhythmic therapy.  N Engl J Med 303:607, 1980.

10. Graboys TB, Lown B, Podrid PJ, et al.:  Long-term survival of patients with malignant ventricular arrhythmia treated with antiarrhythmic drugs.  Am J Cardiol 50:437, 1982.

11. Vlay SC, Kallman CH, Reid PR:  Prognostic assessment of survivors of ventricular tachycardia and ventricular fibrillation with ambulatory monitoring.  Am J Cardiol 54:87, 1984.

12. Morganroth J, Michelson EL, Horowitz LN, et al.:  Limitations of routine long-term electrocardiographic monitoring to assess ventricular ectopic frequency.  Circulation 58:408, 1978.

13. Myerburg RJ, Kessler KM, Kien I, et al.:  Relationship between plasma levels of procainamide, suppression of premature ventricular complexes and prevention of recurrent ventricular tachycardia. Circulation 64:280, 1981.

14. Clark PI, Glasser SP, Spoto E Jr, et al.:  Arrhythmias detected by ambulatory monitoring:  Lack of correlation with symptoms of dizziness and syncope.  Chest 77:722, 1980.

15. McGovern B, DiMarco JP, Garan H, et al.:  New concepts in the management of ventricular arrhythmias and sudden death.  Curr Probl Cardiol 7:6, 1983.

16. Hiss RG, Lamb LE:  Electrocardiographic findings in 122,043 individuals.  Circulation 25:947, 1962.

17. Brodsky M, Wu D, Denes P, et al.:  Arrhythmias documented by 24 hour continuous electrocardiographic monitoring in 50 male medical studies without apparent heart disease.  Am J Cardiol 39:390, 1977.

18. Lown B, Wolf M:  Approaches to sudden death from coronary heart disease.  Circulation 44:130, 1971.

19. The Coronary Drug Project Research Group:  Prognostic importance of premature beats following myocardial infarction.  Experience in the Coronary Drug Project.  JAMA 223:1116, 1973.

20. Schulze RA, Strauss HW, Pitt B:  Sudden death in the year following myocardial infarction: Relation to ventricular premature contractions in the late hospital phase and left ventricular ejection fraction.  Am J Med 62:192, 1977.

21. Packer M:  Sudden unexpected death in patients with congestive heart failure:  A second frontier.  Circulation 72:681, 1985.

22. Kennedy HL, Whitlock JA, Sprague MK, et al.:  Long-term follow-up of asymptomatic healthy subjects with frequent and complex ventricular ectopy.  N Engl J Med 312:193, 1985

23. Podrid PJ, Lown B, Graboys TB, et al.: Use of short-term drug testing as part of a systematic approach for evaluation of antiarrhythmic drugs.  Circulation 73:II-81, 1986.

24. Bigger JT, Reiffel JA, Livelli FD, et al.:  Sensitivity, specificity, and reproducibility of programmed ventricular stimulation.  Circulation 73:II-73, 1986.

25. Josephson ME, Horowitz LN, Harken AH:  Surgery for recurrent ventricular tachycardia associated with coronary artery disease: The role of endocardial resection.  Ann NY Acad Sci 382:381, 1982.

26. Stevenson WG, Brugada P, Waldecker B, et al.:  Clinical, angiographic, and electrophysiologic findings in patients with aborted sudden death as compared with patients with sustained ventricular tachycardia after myocardial infarction.  Circulation 71:1146, 1985.

27. Waspe LE, Seinfeld D, Ferrick A, et al.:  Prediction of sudden death and spontaneous ventricular tachycardia in survivors of complicated myocardial infarction:  Value of the response to programmed stimulation using a maximum of three ventricular extrastimuli.  J Am Coll Cardiol 5:1292, 1985.

28. Beta-blocker Heart Attack Trial Research Group:  A randomized trial of propranolol in patients with acute myocardial infarction.  I. Mortality results.  JAMA 247:1707, 1982.

29. Norwegian Multicenter Study Group:  Timolol-induced reduction in mortality and reinfarction in patients surviving acute myocardial infarction.  N Engl J Med 304:801, 1981.

30. Ryden L, Ariniego R, Arnman K, et al.:  A double-blind trial of metoprolol in acute myocardial infarction.  Effects on ventricular tachyarrhythmias.  N Engl J Med 308:614, 1983.

# Chapter 16

# Cardiopulmonary Resuscitation

### INITIAL MANAGEMENT

The house officer will most frequently encounter cardiopulmonary arrest in the hospitalized patient with known or suspected cardiac disease or other severe underlying illness. When cardiopulmonary arrest is recognized, a rapid initial assessment of the setting in which it occurred should be made as the A-B-C's of basic life support are set in motion:

A. **Airway** -- open and clear airway.
B. **Breathing** -- ventilate mouth-to-mouth or with a bag-valve-mask device.
C. **Circulation** -- chest compression.

**Only after basic life support has been initiated should attention be directed to advanced life support,** i.e., intravenous drug therapy, defibrillation, cardiac pacing, etc. Once cardiopulmonary resuscitation (CPR) has been initiated, the effectiveness of artificial circulation should be assessed by frequent palpation of the carotid or femoral arteries. However, it should be remembered that **the amplitude of the palpated pulse is not a direct reflection of cardiac output or systemic perfusion during closed-chest CPR.** In the hospital setting, the effectiveness of artificial ventilation should be assessed with frequent arterial blood gas analysis. Chest compression should be continued until a palpable arterial pulse is consistently produced by spontaneous cardiac contractions or until a decision is made to cease resuscitative efforts.

In certain clinical settings, **definitive therapy** can and should be administered as soon as possible after the recognition of cardiopulmonary arrest. **Ventricular fibrillation** (VF) is the first encountered rhythm in about 50% of in-hospital cardiac arrests. Electrical defibrillation is the definitive therapy. If the onset of VF is witnessed or if VF is identified in a patient who has been in cardiac arrest for less than 2 min, immediate countershock (200-300 W/sec) should be performed if a defibrillator is readily available(1). Establishing an intravenous line or administering medications is not the first priority in this situation. If countershock restores a viable rhythm and palpable pulse, vital organ perfusion will be significantly better than that achieved with conventional CPR.

If the clinical setting is sudden cardiovascular collapse and loss of consciousness during a procedure (thoracentesis, arterial puncture, induction of anesthesia, etc.), a **vasovagal reaction** should be suspected. Hemodynamic studies indicate that such reactions are characterized by a decrease in heart rate, cardiac output, peripheral vascular resistance, and arterial pressure and are produced by a generalized inhibition of sympathetic tone with a relative increase in vagal (parasympathetic) activity(2).    Atropine, 1.0–4.0 mg intravenously, should be administered immediately after the A-B-C's of basic life support have been instituted.    Vasopressors (high-dose dopamine, >20 mcg/kg/min, or norepinephrine), epinephrine, and intravenous fluids may also be utilized if atropine does not significantly improve systemic perfusion.

## ASSESSMENT

After the institution of basic cardiac life support, during the initial phase of advanced life support, or following successful resuscitation, a more thorough assessment of the patient should be undertaken.   If cardiac arrest occurred out-of-hospital, an abbreviated history should be obtained from the victim's family or friends. **Important physical findings which may suggest causes for the cardiopulmonary arrest or reasons for failure of conventional resuscitation measures include:**

1.  Evidence of overt trauma to head, neck, chest, or abdomen.

2.  Flat neck veins during resuscitation suggests hypovolemia.

3.  Markedly distended neck veins during or following resuscitation suggest cardiac tamponade, pulmonary embolism, or severe biventricular failure.

4.  Inequality of breath sounds may indicate malposition of the endotracheal tube (intubation of right mainstem bronchus), pneumothorax, hemo- or hydrothorax, and/or large airway obstruction (aspiration).

5.  Abdominal distension suggests gastric insufflation from artificial ventilation, ruptured abdominal aortic aneurysm, and/or hemoperitoneum from splenic or hepatic trauma.

6.  Peripheral edema may be an indication of chronic congestive heart failure.   Inequality of calf size or other clinical findings of deep vein thrombosis may be indicative of an antecedent pulmonary or paradoxical embolism.

7.  Grossly bloody or melanotic stools on rectal examination suggests gastrointestinal bleeding and hypovolemia.

8.  Unilateral pupil dilatation and unresponsiveness are indicative of a catastrophic central nervous system (CNS) event. Bilaterally dilated and fixed pupils may be due to inadequate perfusion during CPR or the result of atropine used during the resuscitative attempt.

## CARDIAC RHYTHM DISTURBANCES ENCOUNTERED IN CARDIOPULMONARY ARREST:   A BASIC APPROACH TO MANAGEMENT

**VF is the first rhythm encountered in the majority of arrests** and can be converted to a perfusing supraventricular rhythm in approximately 20-30% of patients. It may be precipitated by ischemia, hypoxemia, and acid-base or electrolyte imbalances which may alter automaticity or conduction, i.e., facilitate re-entry. Less than 5% of arrests due to primary bradycardia or asystole are successfully resuscitated[3,4]. **Causes of primary bradycardic/asystolic arrest include**[5]:

1.  Bradycardia following inferior myocardial infarction (MI).

2.  Heart block following anterior MI.

3.  Asystole following MI.

4.  Myocardial rupture.

5.  Drug-induced asystole or malignant bradycardia.

6.  Sudden bradycardic/asystolic cardiac arrest.

Asystole or a nonperfusing (pulseless) spontaneous rhythm frequently follows countershock of VF.   Such an outcome is nearly always fatal[6,7].

If the onset of VF is witnessed or is documented in a patient who has been in cardiac arrest for less than 2 min, immediate countershock with 200-300 W/sec is recommended.   If VF is identified in a patient in cardiac arrest of indeterminate duration, the A-B-C's of basic life support should be initiated and continued for 2 min before countershock is attempted. Countershock is usually followed by one of four outcomes:

1.  A perfusing supraventricular rhythm.

2.  Bradycardia (sinus, nodal, or idioventricular), with or without arterial pulsations.

3.  Persistent ventricular fibrillation.

4.  Asystole.

Generally accepted therapy for each of these situations is outlined below.

## SUPRAVENTRICULAR RHYTHM

1.  Maintain airway and oxygenation.

2.  Correct acid-base disturbances as guided by arterial blood gas analysis.

3.  **Lidocaine,** 75 mg slow IV bolus, followed by an infusion at a rate of 2 mg/min (lidocaine therapy is not likely to affect the supraventricular rhythm, but is designed to minimize the possibility of recurrent VF). If ventricular ectopy appears or persists, additional boluses of 50 mg can be given at 5-minute intervals to a total bolus dose of 225 mg. The constant infusion rate can also be increased but should not exceed 4 mg/min. The bolus dose or infusion rate should be decreased by 50% in patients with left ventricular (LV) failure or hepatic dysfunction.

4.  If perfusion appears inadequate, consider **volume replacement** ("fluid challenge"), **vasopressors,** or **cardioversion** if a rapid tachyarrhythmia is present.

## BRADYARRHYTHMIA

1.  Maintain airway and oxygenation.

2.  Correct acid-base disturbances as guided by arterial blood gas analysis.

3.  Administer **atropine,** 1.0-2.0 mg intravenously in 0.5-mg increments to increase the heart rate to 50 or more beats/min.

4.  If atropine is ineffective and perfusion inadequate, **isoproterenol** (Isuprel) may be administered as a constant infusion at a rate of 2-20 mcg/min and titrated to the heart rate and rhythm response. However, **isoproterenol may decrease peripheral arterial tone and decrease myocardial blood flow.** Epinephrine, which has both alpha- and beta-adrenergic effects, may be more efficacious.

    Bradycardia and hypotension caused by excessive parasympathetic tone may not respond to catecholamines unless cholinergic blockade is initially achieved with atropine(8).

5.  If there is no significant hemodynamic response to atropine or adrenergic agonists, **cardiac pacing** should be attempted. Transvenous, transthoracic, or transcutaneous techniques are available.

## PERSISTENT VENTRICULAR FIBRILLATION

1. Immediately countershock a second time with 200-300 W/sec.

2. Countershock a third time with 360-400 W/sec.

3. If ineffective, i.e., persistent VF, continue CPR.

4. Administer **epinephrine**, 0.5-1.0 mg (5-10 ml of a 1:10,000 solution), and **sodium bicarbonate** if indicated by arterial blood gas analysis.

5. Countershock a fourth time with 360-400 W/sec.

6. If ineffective, assess adequacy of ventilation and chest compression. **Repeat epinephrine**, 0.5-1.0 mg intravenously, or **administer lidocaine**, 75-100 mg intravenously. After approximately 2 min of continued CPR, countershock should again be attempted with 360-400 W/sec.

7. If ineffective, assess adequacy of ventilation and chest compression. Assess acid-base status and administer sodium bicarbonate as indicated from the calculated base deficit. **Repeat lidocaine**, 75-100 mg IV bolus. **Procainamide**, 10-12 mg/kg over 10-20 min, or **bretylium**, 5-10 mg/kg over 5 min, can also be used.

8. After lidocaine, procainamide, or bretylium has been given, allow 2 min for circulation/distribution with CPR, then countershock with 360-400 W/sec.

9. In patients with **torsades de pointes** and refractory or recurrent VF, IV magnesium sulfate or isoproterenol may be of value(9).

   Persistent or refractory VF is nearly always fatal. There are no clinically relevant studies to suggest that one antiarrhythmic drug is superior in this situation. Likewise, use of anterior-posterior defibrillator paddle placement after failed sternal-apical placement is of unproven value.

## ASYSTOLE

1. Continue CPR.

2. Administer **atropine** 1 mg IV, or **epinephrine** 1 mg IV.

3. If no electrical activity is noted, assess acid-base status and administer sodium bicarbonate as indicated. **Isoproterenol and calcium chloride are of unproven value** in this setting, may be detrimental, and are not recommended(10,11).

5.  If no electrical activity is noted, **cardiac pacing** may be attempted but is unlikely to be successful.

## DRUG THERAPY DURING CPR

### ATROPINE

Atropine sulfate is a parasympatholytic drug.  Its direct cardiac vagolytic action accelerates the rate of discharge of the sinus node and may improve atrioventricular conduction.  Its effects on parasympathetic tone may allow circulating endogenous catecholamines to exert their maximum effects and stimulate the release of additional catecholamines(8).  Atropine is **most frequently used to treat** severe sinus bradycardia when associated with hypotension or frequent ventricular escape beats.  It may also be used to treat high degree-atrioventricular block, slow idioventricular rates, and asystole.

### Dose

The parasympathetic blocking dose of atropine is approximately 0.05 mg/kg of body weight, or 3.5–4.0 mg for an adult.  It is better to err on the side of "overdosage" in circulatory arrest than to permit the vagal "brakes" to render intrinsic or extrinsic catecholamines ineffective. **When treating symptomatic sinus bradycardia,** atropine should be given in 0.5-mg increments at 5-min intervals until the desired response is achieved, or a total dose of 2 mg is given.

### EPINEPHRINE

Epinephrine is one of the most frequently used drugs during advanced cardiac life support.  Its use is based upon both its peripheral alpha-adrenergic effects and cardiac beta-agonist actions. Peripheral vascular effects result in an increased myocardial perfusion pressure and redistribution of available blood flow to vital organs during CPR(10,12). Increased automaticity and positive inotropic effect result from beta-receptor stimulation.  **Epinephrine is recommended** in pulseless brady-arrhythmias, asystole, and for the management of VF which does not respond to electrical countershock.

### Dose

The recommended dose of epinephrine is 0.5 to 1.0 mg (5–10 ml of a 1:10,000 solution) given intravenously.  Repeated 0.5–1.0-mg doses of epinephrine may be administered at 5-min intervals as needed.  A higher dose may be required if the tracheobronchial route of administration is used(13).  Epinephrine can also be administered via constant IV infusion.

## SODIUM BICARBONATE

Limited systemic perfusion and oxygen delivery during cardio-pulmonary arrest and CPR result in the production of lactic acid, the end product of anaerobic metabolism. Sodium bicarbonate is administered during CPR to treat the resultant metabolic acidosis. **Sodium bicarbonate should not be administered indiscriminately;** when used in excess, metabolic alkalosis, hypernatremia, and hyperosmolarity may result(14,15). In addition, sodium bicarbonate administration will raise $PCO_2$, which may profoundly affect myocardial contractility.

### Dose

In the hospital setting, **bicarbonate dose should be guided by arterial blood gas and pH determinations** and assessment of base deficit using standard formulae as guidelines:

pH decrease of 0.15 units = base deficit of 10 mEq/L.

Dose of bicarbonate (mEq) = base deficit (mEq/L) x
body weight (kg) x 0.25
(the bicarbonate "space")

Sudden and total corrections may be hazardous. It is recommended that 50% of the calculated dose be given initially with subsequent doses determined by reassessment of acid-base status. **Sodium bicarbonate should not be used to treat respiratory acidosis.**

## ISOPROTERENOL

Isoproterenol is a synthetic sympathomimetic amine with nearly pure beta-adrenergic agonist activity. Intravenous administration results in an increase in heart rate, an increase in myocardial contractility, and a decrease in peripheral vascular resistance. However, an imbalance between cardiac and peripheral vascular effects may result in a decrease in myocardial perfusion pressure despite an increase in cardiac output. The increase in myocardial oxygen demand occasioned by an increased heart rate and a heightened contractile state may not be met with an increase in myocardial oxygen delivery. During CPR, isoproterenol is most commonly used to treat bradyarrhythmias unresponsive to atropine, heart block, and asystole. Its efficacy in these settings is unproven. **Experimental observations suggest that this agent is of limited value and may be detrimental.**

### Dose

Isoproterenol is usually administered as a constant infusion at a rate of 2-20 mcg/min. One milligram of isoproterenol in 250 ml of 5% dextrose provides a concentration of 4 mcg/ml. Isoproterenol may also be given as 2-5 mcg boluses to a total dose of 20 mcg.

## CALCIUM CHLORIDE

The calcium ion is known to have a positive effect upon the contractile state of the myocardium mediated through excitation-contraction coupling. Additional electrophysiologic effects mediated via "slow channels" have also been described(16). The role of slow channel or calcium-mediated responses in the genesis of arrhythmias in the hypoxic myocardium and following reperfusion is presently under active investigation.

Several recent studies indicate that calcium administration during cardiac arrest is of limited value(11,17,18). It is of no value in asystole and of questionable benefit in electromechanical dissociation (EMD). Calcium administration may in fact be detrimental, as intracellular calcium accumulation may play a role in cell death. At present, **calcium use during CPR is recommended only in selected situations**, i.e., cardiac arrest due to hyperkalemia, hypocalcemia, or following use of calcium-blocking agents.

### Dose

Calcium chloride is usually given in a dose of 5 ml of a 10% solution and repeated if necessary in 10 min. The 10% solution contains 1.36 mEq $Ca^{+2}$/100 mg of salt (100 mg of salt = 1.36 mEq of $Ca^{+2}$ = 1 ml). Calcium should never be given in the same intravenous line with bicarbonate, since it will precipitate.

## LIDOCAINE

Lidocaine is currently the drug of choice for the management of ventricular ectopy in the setting of cardiopulmonary arrest. Its effect on spontaneous phase 4 depolarization, conduction velocity in the Purkinje network, and dispersion of recovery of excitability (refractory period) combine to make it an effective agent in the management of ventricular arrhythmias due to re-entry or ectopic, automatic foci. It is recommended for use in the treatment of ventricular extrasystoles, ventricular tachycardia, and ventricular fibrillation when countershock has failed. It should also be administered following successful defibrillation.

### Dose

Lidocaine is administered as a slow intravenous bolus (1 mg/kg of body weight) to achieve a therapeutic blood level followed by a constant infusion at a rate of 1-4 mg/min using a controlled infusion device(19). If ventricular ectopy persists after the initial bolus, additional slow 50-mg boluses may be given every 5 min until the arrhythmia is suppressed or until 225 mg has been given(20). After each additional bolus, the constant infusion rate should be increased by 1 mg/min to a maximum of 4 mg/min.  The bolus dose should be decreased by 50% in the presence of reduced cardiac output, liver dysfunction, or in patients over 65 years of age.

## BRETYLIUM

Bretylium tosylate is a second-line antiarrhythmic drug used in the treatment of ventricular tachycardia or ventricular fibrillation which is refractory to other forms of therapy. Following intravenous injection, bretylium has been shown to release tissue catecholamines and later produce postganglionic adrenergic blockage(21). The drug also has direct cardiac effects which are incompletely defined. Its dominant electrophysiologic effect is uniform prolongation of action potential duration. In the clinical setting of cardiac arrest, this agent has not been convincingly shown to be superior to lidocaine(22).

### Dose

In refractory VF, bretylium is given as a 5-mg/kg intravenous bolus. Countershock may be attempted 2-5 min later. If VF persists, 10 mg/kg may be given and repeated at 15-30 min intervals to a maximum dose of 30 mg/kg.

## SPECIAL PROBLEMS ENCOUNTERED DURING CARDIOPULMONARY RESUSCITATION

1. **Persistent hypoxemia despite high concentrations of inspired oxygen.  Consider:**

   - Endotracheal tube in right mainstem bronchus or esophagus.

   - Aspiration, pneumonia, pulmonary edema.

   - Pneumothorax.

   - Pulmonary embolus.

   - Gastric distension.

2. **Electromechanical dissociation.  Consider**(23):

   - Decreased preload (hypovolemia)--look for tachycardia with a low central venous pressure.

   - Cardiac tamponade--look for tachycardia with an elevated central venous pressure.

   - Outflow obstruction (i.e., pulmonary embolus)--look for tachycardia with an elevated central venous pressure.

- Myocardial depression—look for tachycardia with an elevated central venous pressure.

3. **Open chest cardiac massage—When should it be used(24)?**

- Cardiopulmonary arrest associated with or following overt trauma (closed or penetrating) to the chest or abdomen. Open chest massage will allow direct evaluation of possible cardiac tamponade, facilitate control of intrathoracic bleeding, and permit "cross-clamping" of the descending thoracic aorta if indicated.

- In patients with flail chests.

- In suspected cardiac tamponade.

- If massive air embolism is suspected, open chest massage permits direct air aspiration from the right heart.

- If ruptured abdominal aortic aneurysm is suspected, cross-clamping of the descending aorta may be performed if indicated.

- Cardiopulmonary arrest occurring during intrathoracic surgical procedures.

- In cardiopulmonary arrest due to severe hypothermia, the direct approach will allow saline rewarming of the heart.

- In patients with prosthetic cardiac valves.

- If external defibrillation proves ineffective and internal paddles are available.

4. **Intracardiac drug administration:**

The intracardiac route for direct administration should be avoided unless it is not possible to achieve a reliable access route in a peripheral or central vein.

5. **Termination of CPR:**

At present there are no well defined guidelines to aid the physician in deciding when to cease resuscitative efforts. It is difficult to apply the usual clinical criteria of brain death to the cardiac arrest victim who is receiving seemingly effective CPR. The decision to cease resuscitative efforts should be based upon the failure of properly applied basic and advance cardiac life support to re-establish effective cardiac function(1). Utilizing these criteria will eliminate speculation as to brain viability.

## REFERENCES

1. Standards and guidelines for cardiopulmonary resuscitation (CPR) and emergency cardiac care (ECC). JAMA 255:2841, 1986.

2. Glick G, Yu PN: Hemodynamic changes during spontaneous vasovagal reactions. Am J Cardiol 38:268,1963.

3. Bedell SE, Delbanco TL, Cook EF, et al.: Survival after cardiopulmonary resuscitation in the hospital. N Engl J Med 309:569,1983.

4. Roth R, Steward RD, Rodgers K, et al.: Out-of-hospital cardiac arrest. Factors associated with survival. Ann Emerg Med 13:237, 1984.

5. Greenberg HM: Bradycardia at onset of sudden death: Potential mechanisms. Ann NY Acad Sci 427:241, 1984.

6. Weaver WD, Cobb LA, Dennis D, et al.: Amplitude of ventricular fibrillation waveform and outcome after cardiac arrest. Ann Intern Med 102:53, 1985.

7. Warner LL, Hoffman JR, Baraff LJ: Prognostic significance of field response in out-of-hospital ventricular fibrillation. Chest 87:22, 1985.

8. Brown DC, Lewis AJ, Criley JM: Asystole and its treatment: The possible role of the parasympathetic nervous system in cardiac arrest. Journal of the American College of Emergency Physicians 8:448, 1979.

9. Keren A, Tzivoni D, Gavish D, et al.: Etiology, warning signs and therapy of torsade de pointes. A study of 10 patients. Circulation 64:1167, 1981.

10. Niemann JT, Haynes K, Garner D, et al.: Postcountershock pulseless rhythms: Response to CPR, immediate cardiac pacing, and adrenergic agonists. Ann Emerg Med 15:112, 1986.

11. Donovan PJ, Propp DA: Calcium and its role in cardiac arrest: Understanding the controversy. J Emerg Med 3:105, 1985.

12. Michael JR, Guerci AD, Koehler RC, et al.: Mechanisms by which epinephrine augments cerebral and myocardial perfusion during cardiopulmonary resuscitation in dogs. Circulation 69:822, 1984.

13. Ralston SH, Tacker WA, Showen L, et al.: Endotracheal versus intravenous epinephrine during electromechanical dissociation with CPR in dogs. Ann Emerg Med 11:1044, 1985.

14. Bishop RL, Weisfeldt ML:  Sodium bicarbonate administration during cardiac arrest:  Effect on arterial pH, pCO2, and osmolality.  JAMA 235:506, 1976.

15. Niemann JT, Rosborough JP:  Effects of acidemia and sodium bicarbonate therapy in advanced cardiac life support.  Ann Emerg Med 13:781, 1984.

16. Bailey JC, Elharrar V, Zipes DP:  Slow-channel depolarization: Mechanism and control of arrhythmias.  Ann Rev Med 29:417, 1978.

17. Harrison EE, Amey BD:  The use of calcium in cardiac resuscitation.  Am J Emerg Med 3:267, 1983.

18. Stueven HA, Thompson BM, Aprahamian C, et al.:  Calcium chloride: Reassessment of use in asystole.  Ann Emerg Med 13:820, 1984.

19. Harrison DC:  Practical guidelines for the use of lidocaine.  JAMA 233:1202, 1975.

20. Wyman MG, Lalka D, Hammersmith L, et al.:  Multiple bolus technique for lidocaine administration during the first hours of an acute myocardial infarction.  Am J Cardiol 41:313, 1978.

21. Koch-Weser J:  Drug therapy:  Bretylium.  N Engl J Med 300:473, 1979.

22. Haynes RE, Chinn TL, Copass MK, et al.:  Comparison of bretylium tosylate and lidocaine in management of out-of-hospital ventricular fibrillation.  Am J Cardiol 48:353, 1981.

23. Friedman HS:  Diagnostic considerations in electro-mechanical dissociation.  Am J Cardiol 38:448, 1979.

24. Stephenson HE:  Pathophysiologic considerations that warrant open-chest cardiac resuscitation.  Crit Care Med 8:185, 1980.

# Chapter 17

# Artificial
# Cardiac Pacemakers

Implantable cardiac pacemakers were first used in the treatment of bradyarrhythmias in the late 1950s. The first pacemakers were bulky, fixed-rate and incapable of sensing the intrinsic rhythm (competitive or asynchronous), and often lasted <1 year. Contemporary pacemakers are engineering masterpieces; they are compact and lightweight, are capable of sensing and pacing in both the right atrium and ventricle, can last 10 years or longer, and are externally programmable(1,2).

There are many different types of pacemakers available to the clinician. However, **all pacemakers are composed of three basic elements:** 1) the power source or battery, 2) the electronic circuitry, and 3) the lead system that connects the pulse generator to the heart.

## POWER SOURCES

All pacemakers have a battery that supplies energy to stimulate the heart, as well as to maintain the circuitry needed to sense properly and to regulate the timing of electrical stimuli. The major source of energy drain is pacing (electrical discharge). **External, temporary pacemakers use standard household-type alkaline or mercury batteries.** Implantable pacemakers originally used mercury-zinc batteries that were bulky and had a short life span. Externally rechargeable batteries were later introduced but were plagued by physician and patient fears that the patient would forget to recharge the battery on a monthly basis. Nuclear-powered batteries had the theoretical advantage of an extremely long life span, but regulatory agencies have made their use cumbersome and difficult for physicians. In the 1970s, lithium batteries were introduced, and **almost all currently implanted permanent pacemakers are lithium powered.** They offer the advantages of both light weight and long life. Current estimates indicate that some lithium powered pacemakers may last 15 to 20 years. Clinical data have shown that approximately 75% of lithium-powered pacemakers are still functioning after 7 years(3). **This has almost eliminated sudden power depletion as a cause of permanent pacemaker failure.**

## PACEMAKER LEADS

Pacemaker leads can be placed either epicardially, such as at the time of open heart surgery, or endocardially using transvenous techniques. **Most permanent pacemakers (90%) now use endocardial leads that are positioned in the heart using a subclavian or cephalic vein approach.** Pacemaker leads, like the battery sources, have undergone major technical improvements over the years. Innovations have included resilient plastic insulation surrounding the electrodes that reduces the chance of lead fracture or breakage. Endocardial leads have also been designed to "actively" fixate to the atrial or ventricular endocardial surface using tined or screw-in tips(4). Atrial leads can be preshaped into a "J" to allow proper and more stable positioning in the atrial appendage.

**Pacemaker leads can be either bipolar or unipolar in configuration.** Bipolar endocardial leads have both the negative (distal) and positive (proximal) leads within the heart (usually only 1-2 cm apart). Unipolar leads have the negative lead in contact with the endocardial surface, and the positive pole is the metallic casing of the pulse generator. Unipolar leads theoretically provide better sensing, but this has not been of major importance in clinical studies. Unipolar leads, however, do tend to oversense noncardiac electrical activity such as muscle artifact (myopotentials) or electromagnetic interference.

## PACEMAKER MODALITIES

**A pacemaker has two basic functions:** 1) to electrically stimulate the heart and 2) to sense intrinsic cardiac electrical activity. The pacemaker will deliver an electrical stimulus to either the atrium or ventricle if it does not recognize (sense) any intrinsic electrical activity from that chamber after a programmed interval. If it does recognize or sense the P wave (atrium) or QRS (ventricle), the pacemaker will inhibit or reset the output of the pacemaker to prevent "competition" with the underlying rhythm.

**A classification code** has been developed to serve as a shorthand method of identifying in which chamber(s) a pacemaker is functioning (Table 17.1). **A five-letter code identifies all the major functions of the pacemaker**(5). The first and second letters denote which chamber(s) the pacemaker paces and senses, respectively. The third letter shows the mode of response of the pacemaker (I=inhibited or "reset"; T=triggered or discharged). The fourth and fifth letters are optional and are often not used when referring to a type of pacemaker. Examples of types of pacemakers using the code include: **DVI**--pacing in both the atria and ventricle but sensing only in the ventricle in the inhibited mode; **AAT**--sensing and pacing only in the atria in the triggered mode. The triggered mode is usually programmed to detect sensing problems since a pacing artifact is discharged within each sensed cardiac event; **DDD**--pacing and sensing in both the atria and ventricle and in the atrial tracking mode of response; **VVI**--ventricular pacing and sensing in the inhibited mode.

Table 17.1
Five-Letter Pacemaker Code

| PACE | SENSE | MODE | PROGRAMMABILITY* | TACHYCARDIA* |
|------|-------|------|------------------|--------------|
| A=Atrium | A=Atrium | I=Inhibited | P=Programmable rate or output only | E=Externally activated |
| V=Ventricle | V=Ventricle | T=Triggered | | B=Burst |
| D=Dual | D=Dual | D=Dual | M=Multiprogrammable | S=Scanning |
| | O=None | O=Asynchronous | O=None | O=None |

*Optional letter

Originally, pacemakers were discharged at a fixed rate and had no sensing circuit (asynchronous)(AOO or VOO). This modality is now rarely used. However, a magnet placed over a pulse generator will temporarily convert most pacemakers to an asynchronous mode (e.g., a VVI pacemaker becomes VOO). This technique is useful to demonstrate that the pacemaker is still capable of pacing and capturing if a patient's intrinsic rhythm is inhibiting the pacemaker.

**Dual chamber pacemakers** came into wider use in the late 1970s. This technological advance was made possible because of more stable atrial leads and the use of microprocessor-based multiprogrammable pulse generators. Dual chamber pacemakers, such as DDD pacemakers, have three major advantages over ventricular pacemakers(2):

1. The proper timing of atrial contraction is maintained prior to ventricular contraction. Atrial contribution to ventricular filling may augment cardiac output by 10-25%.

2. Sinus control over ventricular rate is maintained. Therefore, when the sinus rate increases with exertion, the ventricular pacing rate will increase, as opposed to the single rate response of a single chamber pacemaker(6,7). The dual chamber pacemaker still will pace the atrium at a minimal programmed rate in response to bradycardia.

3. Occasionally, patients will be symptomatic with dizziness or near syncope with VVI pacing. This is known as the "pacemaker syndrome" and can often be alleviated by using a dual chamber pacemaker(8).

**Table 17.2**
**Ventricular Versus Dual Chamber Pacing**(2)

**Ventricular pacing (VVI) indicated:**

1. For patients in whom pacing is used only to treat transient symptomatic bradyarrhythmias (e.g., sick sinus syndrome).

2. For patients in atrial fibrillation or flutter or with poorly contracting atria.

3. For patients in whom there is no anticipated significant hemodynamic benefit from atrial contraction.

4. For "sustenance" pacing in the inactive invalid or inactive institutionalized elderly in whom the added cost of a dual chamber device may not be worthwhile or beneficial.

**Dual chamber pacing indicated when the clinician wishes to:**

1. Maintain responsiveness of heart rate to increased demand, e.g., exercise.

2. Provide the "booster pump" function of atrial contraction to maximize ventricular function, e.g., patients with CHF in sinus rhythm.

### INDICATIONS FOR TEMPORARY PACEMAKER

Temporary pacemakers are indicated for the treatment of bradycardias that are transient or prior to the insertion of a permanent pacemaker. Transient bradyarrhythmias are most commonly due to drug toxicity (most often digoxin or beta blockers) and acute myocardial infarction. Temporary pacing may also be used prophylactically in patients with left bundle branch block prior to insertion of a pulmonary artery catheter.

**Indications for prophylactic temporary pacing during an acute myocardial infarction** are controversial(9). Temporary pacemakers are electively placed in those patients who are **likely** to develop complete heart block as a result of an acute myocardial infarction. Table 17.3 summarizes clinical data which suggest a high incidence (>20%) of complete heart block in patients with acute infarction and certain conduction disturbances. Since these patients often have very large anterior infarctions, mortality remains high despite prophylactic demand pacing, since death is most often due to pump failure rather than arrhythmias.

Table 17.3
Prophylactic Pacing in Acute Myocardial Infarction

| INDICATED | NOT INDICATED | CONTROVERSIAL |
|---|---|---|
| 1)  Mobitz II AV block | 1) 1st degree AV block | 1) New LBBB |
| 2)  Complete AV block | 2) Wenckebach 2nd degree AV block | 2) New RBBB in IMI |
| 3)  New RBBB in AMI | 3) Old LBBB | |
| 4)  RBBB + LAFB | 4) Old RBBB | |
| 5)  RBBB + LPFB | | |
| 6)  LBBB + 1st degree AV block | | |
| 7)  Symptomatic bradycardia | | |

-----

```
AV   = Atrioventricular
LBBB = Left bundle branch block
RBBB = Right bundle branch block
LAFB = Left anterior fascicular block
LPFB = Left posterior fascicular block
AMI  = Anterior myocardial infarction
IMI  = Inferior myocardial infarction
```

## INDICATIONS FOR PERMANENT PACEMAKER

The indications for permanent pacemaker insertion are based on data which suggest that improvement in the quality and length of life can be affected(10)(Table 17.4).  Prior to permanent implantation, a careful search should be made for treatable causes of the arrhythmia or conduction defect, e.g., drug toxicity, electrolyte disturbances, ischemia/infarction, infection, or thyroid disease.   An arrhythmia can be chronic or intermittent.  However, a thorough attempt should be made to directly correlate symptoms due to the rhythm disorder in patients who have only intermittent disturbances.  Prolonged ambulatory (Holter) monitoring may be necessary.

**Table 17.4**
**Indications for Permanent Pacemaker**

|  | ALWAYS | CONTROVERSIAL | NOT INDICATED |
|---|---|---|---|
| AV BLOCK | Symptomatic CHB<br>Symptomatic 2AVB | Asymptomatic CHB<br>Asymptomatic 1AVB | 1AVB |
| AFTER MI | Persistent 2AVB or CHB | Persistent 1AVB + RBBB | Transient AVB |
| CHRONIC BBB | Bifascicular block with<br>symptomatic AV block | Bifascicular block with<br>asymptomatic AV block | Fascicular<br>block |
| SINUS NODE | Symptomatic bradycardia | Asymptomatic brady-<br>cardia with heart<br>rate of <40 | Asymptomatic<br>bradycardia |

-----
AVB  = Atrioventricular block
CHB  = Complete heart block
1AVB = First degree heart block
2AVB = Second degree heart block
RBBB = Right bundle branch block
BBB  = Bundle branch block

## PACEMAKER PROGRAMMABILITY

Electronic circuitry in pacemakers has advanced in the past several years to allow almost complete external control of pacemaker function. Almost all pacemakers implanted today have some programmability(2,11). Table 17.5 lists features that can be programmed in some pacemakers. Reprogramming is performed using sophisticated devices placed on the skin over the pacemaker power source.

**Table 17.5**
**Programmable Features in Permanent Pacemakers**

MODE

RATE = Lower limit
       Upper limit*

ENERGY OUTPUT = Voltage or pulse width
SENSITIVITY
ATRIOVENTRICULAR INTERVAL ("electronic PR interval")*
REFRACTORY PERIOD
HYSTERESIS
UNIPOLAR/BIPOLAR

*Dual chamber pacemakers

Programming has obvious benefits in allowing the physician to change the function of the pacemaker if the physiologic needs or intrinsic rhythm of the patient change with time.  For example, a patient with a dual chamber (DDD) pacemaker develops paroxysms of atrial tachycardia.  The DDD mode could track this fast atrial rate and pace the ventricle at a rapid rate.  The physician could noninvasively stop sensing of atrial electrical activity by reprogramming the pacemaker to VVI or DVI modes, thus preventing reoperation to replace the pacemaker.  Conversely, a right ventricular infarction could acutely raise the threshold of a VVI pacemaker and cause inability to capture.  Increasing the energy output of the pacemaker by increasing the voltage output or pulse width externally could then result in capture of the ventricle again.

## PACEMAKER FOLLOW-UP

It is very important that patients have regular and adequate follow-up once a permanent pacemaker is implanted(12).  The patient should be seen every 3 to 4 weeks for 2 to 3 visits postimplant to check the implant site for infection or erosion and to assess the adequacy of pacing and sensing.  Visits after the initial period should be approximately every 6 months.  At each visit, a 12-lead ECG should be obtained.  Measurement of pacemaker rate and pulse width using either a pacemaker programmer or a hand-held pacemaker analyzer should also be recorded.  **Most pulse generators begin to show signs of battery failure about 2 years prior to absolute failure by gradually increasing the pulse width or decreasing the pacing rate.**  Most pacemaker manufacturers base their recommended replacement time on these values.  Also, the thresholds of pacing and sensing should be periodically checked to determine that they have not appreciably changed and that a margin of safety exists between actual thresholds and programmed values.  Telephonic monitoring of patients is being used more frequently as a method of assessing patients between office visits.

## PACEMAKER MALFUNCTION(13,14)

**Failure to Pace**

Failure to pace means that the pacemaker discharge or spike does not result in capture or a pacemaker spike does not occur at all.  Failure to pace is due to problems either with the lead or problems with the pulse generator.  Lead problems, the most common cause of failure to pace, include lead fracture, lead displacement, myocardial perforation, or lead-pulse generator disconnection.  Occasionally, there may be problems at the lead-myocardial interface that could increase the threshold to capture (drug effects, electrolyte disorders such as hyperkalemia, infarction, or fibrosis).  If a patient is seen on a regular basis, battery depletion is rarely a cause of loss of capture, although failure to pace due to low battery output can occur.  The rarest cause of failure to pace is pulse generator circuitry failure.

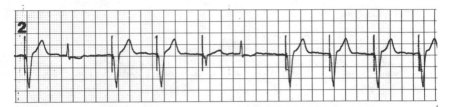

**Figure 17.1 Normal Demand Pacing (VVI mode).**
The patient's spontaneous rhythm is atrial fibrillation with complete heart block and a junctional escape rhythm. The 1st, 3rd, 4th, and 7-10th QRS complexes are wide and preceded by a stimulus artifact (pacemaker spike) and represent normal ventricular capture at a rate of approximately 75/min. The 2nd and 6th QRS complexes are narrow, not preceded by a spike, and represent intrinsic junctional escape beats. In the VVI mode, intrinsic beats are sensed and the pacemaker will not discharge until after a set interval has passed. The 5th QRS complex is preceded by a spike, but the following QRS complex is narrower than other paced beats and has a configuration different from that of beats 2 and 6. This QRS complex represents a fusion beat (a hybrid between normal spontaneous ventricular depolarization and paced beats).

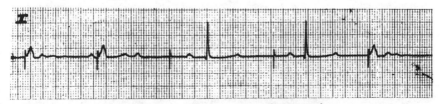

**Figure 17.2 Intermittent Failure to Pace (VVI mode).**
The patient's intrinsic rhythm is complete heart block with atrioventricular dissociation and a junctional escape rhythm. The 1st, 2nd, and 5th pacemaker spikes are followed by ventricular depolarizations

and wide QRS complexes (capture).  The 3rd, 4th, and 6th spikes are not followed by QRS complexes (failure to capture).  The 3rd and 4th QRS complexes are junctional beats preceded by P waves; the PR interval varies (AV dissociation).  The pacemaker discharge rate is 55/min.  Pacemaker malfunction was due to battery depletion in a rechargeable unit set at a rate of 72/min.

## Failure to Sense

Many of the causes of failure to pace, as mentioned above, can also cause failure to sense.  Lead malfunctions are again the most common cause of failure to sense.  Other causes of failure to sense include a decrease in wave form size which may occur in a bundle branch block or infarction.

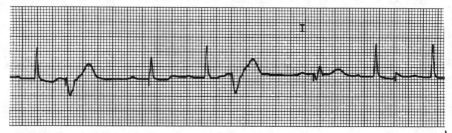

**Figure 17.3  Intermittent Failure to Sense (VVI mode).**
The 2nd and 5th QRS complexes are preceded by a pacemaker spike which occurs during inscription of the T wave of normally conducted intrinsic beats.  The 3rd and 6th QRS complexes are fusion beats following normal sensing and occur at the selected escape rate (54/min).  In this example, intermittent failure to sense resulted in electrical stimulation during the vulnerable period, analogous to the "R-on-T" phenomenon, but did not result in a sustained ventricular arrhythmia.

A pacemaker may remain fixed in an asynchronous mode after a magnet is applied.  When a pacemaker does not recognize a wide, slurred QRS until 40-50 msec of the QRS has elapsed, it may appear that the QRS is not properly sensed since the pacemaker spike occurs in the first 40 msec of the QRS.  This is termed "pseudofusion."

## Oversensing

Occasionally, a pacemaker will sense noncardiac electrical activity rather than an electrical wave form emanating from the heart. An example would be sensing of pectoral muscle myopotentials when the patient moves an upper extremity or performs arm or chest isometric exercise. This results in inhibition of the pacemaker. This could be disastrous if there is no underlying rhythm. Other events that may be inappropriately sensed and cause inhibition include strong electromagnet currents, large and delayed T waves in ventricular sensing pacemakers, and pacing artifact in the opposite chamber in dual chamber pacemakers ("cross-talk").

## Pacemaker-Induced Tachycardia

Dual chamber pacemakers have unique problems as a result of their atrial sensing capability. If a patient with a dual chamber pacemaker in a DDD mode develops an atrial arrhythmia, such as atrial flutter or atrial tachycardia, the ventricle will be paced at that rate up to the programmed upper rate limit. As a result of this problem, dual chamber pacemakers are contraindicated in patients with atrial tacharrhythmias.

Another problem with dual chamber pacemakers (DDD) is known as endless loop tachycardia(15). A ventricular beat could be conducted retrogradely through the atrioventricular (AV) node to depolarize the atrium. This would be sensed by the pacemaker, which has no way of knowing that it was not a sinus beat. After the programmed AV interval, the pacemaker would pace the ventricle. This, in turn, would again be conducted retrogradely to set up a circus or reentrant tachycardia. This can be alleviated by either programming to a DVI mode (eliminate atrial sensing) or increasing the refractory period of the atrial circuitry so that the retrograde P wave falls within the refractory period (therefore, not sensed).

### TACHYCARDIA PACING

Recently, pacemakers have been developed to treat reentrant tachyarrhythmias that are unresponsive to medical therapy(16). Pacemakers can either be activated by the patient using an external transmitter or can be activated automatically when the pacemaker senses the tachycardia. The tachycardia can be terminated by a variety of potential mechanisms: Burst pacing at rates faster than the tachycardia, "underdrive" pacing, or one or more premature stimuli. In addition, devices have been developed to deliver internal shocks to treat either ventricular tachycardia (1 to 2 W/sec) or ventricular fibrillation (up to 25 W/sec) after they are recognized by the pacemaker(17).

## FUTURE DIRECTIONS

Currently available dual chamber pacemakers require an intact sinus node in order to take advantage of the rate responsiveness of these pacemakers. However, many patients have sick sinus syndrome and do not appropriately increase their sinus rate with exertion. Newer prototypes have been developed that will increase ventricular pacing in response to some physiologic parameter other than sinus rate. Examples of physiologic parameters that pacemakers may respond to include muscle activity, temperature, QT interval, respiratory rate, or blood pH.

## REFERENCES

1.  Shively B, Goldschlager N:  Progress in cardiac pacing (Part I). Arch Intern Med 145:2103, 1985.

2.  Shively B, Goldschlager N:  Progress in cardiac pacing (Part II). Arch Intern Med 145:2238, 1985.

3.  Bilitch M, Hauser RG, Goldman BS, et al.:  Performance of cardiac pacemaker pulse generators.  PACE 5:139, 1982.

4.  Furman S, Pannizzo F, Campo I:  Comparison of active and passive adhering leads for endocardial pacing.  PACE 4:78, 1981.

5.  Parsonnet V, Furman S, Smyth NPD:  A revised code for pacemaker identification.  PACE 4:400, 1981.

6.  Kruse I, Arnman K, Conradson T, et al.:  A comparison of acute and long-term hemodynamic effects of ventricular inhibited and atrial synchronous ventricular inhibited pacing.  Circulation 65:846, 1982.

7.  Samet P, Castillo C, Bernstein W:  Hemodynamic consequences of sequential atrioventricular pacing.  Am J Cardiol 21:207, 1968.

8.  Ausubel K, Furman S:  The pacemaker syndrome.  Ann Intern Med 103:420, 1985.

9.  Hindman MC, Wagner GS, Jaro M, et al.:  The clinical significance of bundle branch block complicating acute myocardial infarction.  2. Indications for temporary and permanent pacemaker insertion. Circulation 58:689, 1978.

10. Joint American College of Cardiology/American Heart Association Task Force on Assessment of Cardiovascular Procedures (Subcommittee on Pacemaker Implantation):  Guidelines for permanent cardiac pacemaker implantation, May 1984. J Am Coll Cardiol 4:434, 1984.

11.  Vera Z, Klein RC, Mason DT:  Recent advances in programmable pacemakers.  Consideration of advantages, longevity and future expectations.  Am J Med 66:473, 1979.

12.  Furman S:  Cardiac pacing and pacemakers.  VIII.  The pacemaker follow-up clinic.  Am Heart J 94:795, 1977.

13.  Furman S: Cardiac pacing and pacemakers. VI. Analysis of pacemaker malfunction.  Am Heart J 94:378, 1977.

14.  Furman S:  Pacemaker emergencies.  Med Clin N Am 63:113, 1979.

15.  Luceri RM, Castellanos A, Zaman L, et al.:  The arrhythmias of dual-chamber cardiac pacemakers and their management.  Ann Intern Med 99:354, 1983.

16.  Wiener I:  Pacing techniques in the treatment of tachycardias.  Ann Intern Med 93:326, 1980.

17.  Mirowski M, Reid PR, Mower MM, et al.:  Termination of malignant ventricular arrhythmias with an implanted automatic defibrillator in human beings.  N Engl J Med 303:322, 1980.

# Chapter 18

# Cardiac Surgery

Major advances have been made in the surgical treatment of coronary artery disease (CAD), valvular heart disease, and congenital heart disease. Recent developments in surgical technique, cardiopulmonary bypass technology, cold cardioplegia, newer prosthetic devices, and an increase in surgical experience in the last two decades have accounted for lower morbidity and mortality.

## CORONARY ARTERY SURGERY

In contrast to earlier years when valvular and congenital heart repairs constituted the bulk of surgical cases, coronary artery bypass surgery now accounts for more than 70% of the cardiac surgery done in this country. The principal reasons for considering an operation in CAD are 1) **to improve quality of life** (i.e., relief of angina and improved exercise capacity) and 2) **to improve quantity of life** (increase longevity). **Coronary artery surgery improves the quality of life in the majority of appropriate candidates.** Coronary artery bypass graft surgery will result in complete angina relief in 80% of cases (CABG) and improved but not complete relief in 10%, while 10% will be the same or worse(1). One of the most gratifying consequences of revascularization is that, along with angina relief, the patients usually experience a significant improvement in their ability to perform physical activities. This has been well documented by comparing pre- and postoperative exercise tests(2).

Several large-scale randomized studies of patients with ischemic heart disease have provided important information about **survival with medical and surgical therapy.** The European Coronary Surgery Study (ECSS)(3), the Coronary Artery Surgery Study (CASS)(4), and the Veterans Administration Coronary Artery Bypass Surgery Cooperative Study Group (VACSG)(5) have provided ongoing information over the last 15 years. As these data have been compiled, **it appears that left ventricular (LV) function is the most important determinant of prognosis in patients with CAD.** Other important considerations are the symptomatic status, location of obstructive disease, and the inducibility of ischemia.

The randomized VA study(5) has demonstrated that **patients with left main CAD have improved survival with surgery.** Various authors have reported that the approximate 3-year mortality for significant left main disease is 50% and that surgery (including operative deaths) decreases the mortality in 3 years to approximately 15%(6). **Surgery also improves prognosis for individuals with triple vessel-CAD and left ventricular dysfunction**(7). This trend has been shown in all three of the aforementioned trials and also is seen in the minimally symptomatic subgroup(8). Thus, left ventricular dysfunction has emerged as a major indication for revascularization in markedly symptomatic and minimally symptomatic patients with CAD.

**Survival data between medically and surgically treated patients with triple-vessel disease and normal left ventricular function has yielded conflicting results.** The CASS trial showed no significant difference between these two groups(4), whereas ECSS reported improved survival in the surgical group(3).

A recent study in asymptomatic or mildly symptomatic triple-vessel CAD patients with normal left ventricular function has separated these patient groups into those with no discernible ischemia and those with inducible ischemia (ST depression, decreased ejection fraction on exercise)(8). The group with mild angina, triple-vessel disease, normal LV function on exercise, and no significant ST changes had an excellent prognosis with 100% survival at 4 years. The group with inducible ischemia had only a 71% survival rate over the 4 years.

The number of patients undergoing CABG surgery appears to have plateaued in 1984. Some factors that have tempered the increased use of CABG surgery are major advances in medical treatment, angioplasty, and economic uncertainties. Fewer operations are being done for single-vessel disease and most operations are for markedly symptomatic multivessel CAD.

**Reoperation** is becoming a common occurrence in the 1980s with the leading indication being graft closure(9,10). A surgical problem at the distal anastomosis site is usually the cause of early closure, whereas vein graft atherosclerosis is the most common cause of late graft closure. Evidence suggests that the internal mammary graft shows superior long-term patency when compared to the saphenous vein graft(11). Most reoperations occur after the fifth postoperative year.

**It is important to weigh the benefits and the risks of surgery for each individual case.** In patients with good left ventricular function and satisfactory vessels, the operative mortality should be less than 2% and is less than 1% in many centers. If there is moderate left ventricular dysfunction and smaller or more diseased vessels, mortality rises to 5-7%. If there is severe left ventricular dysfunction, the risk is 10-12%. Morbidity statistics are more difficult to summarize and vary from center to center. There is an approximate 10% risk of stroke, renal failure, or pulmonary embolism. Perioperative myocardial infarction probably occurs in 5-15% of cases, but is usually well tolerated and may be responsible for pain relief in some cases.

## VALVULAR HEART DISEASE

Valvular heart surgery is palliative rather than curative and is generally reserved for significantly symptomatic patients. Certain lesions such as **chronic mitral and aortic regurgitation** may be tolerated for many years without significant functional impairment(12). **The proper timing for operative intervention in either of these types of left ventricular volume overload is often an extremely difficult decision** which requires careful analysis of noninvasive and invasive data(13). Newer echocardiographic and nuclear medicine techniques such as ejection fraction studies at rest and exercise have served as adjuncts in clinical decision making(14).

In mitral regurgitation with a markedly dilated left ventricle (end-diastolic dimension greater than 8.0 cm) and depressed ejection fraction (<45%), mitral valve replacement is not usually associated with improved symptoms and may even lead to an increased mortality. Therefore, surgery is probably not indicated in these patients and medical therapy is preferable. In asymptomatic patients with aortic regurgitation and normal left ventricular function, surgery is not indicated.

Certain valvular lesions have natural histories which can be markedly improved with successful surgery. The average time of survival of patients with **aortic stenosis** is two years after the onset of congestive heart failure, three years with syncope, and five years with angina(12). Operative mortality for valve replacement is less than 5%. After successful repair, patients usually have dramatic improvement in symptoms and the annual mortality falls to less than 5% per year. **Acute insufficiency of the aortic or mitral valve** will often begin precipitously and result in a medical emergency. After initial medical stabilization, the patient may require valve replacement. Along with trauma, valve disruption due to myxomatous changes, dissection, and endocarditis continue to be important etiological factors. Early valve replacement is essential when congestive heart failure or recurrent systemic emboli complicate endocarditis(14).

Many types of **valvular prosthesis** are available(15). The prototype of the ball-and-cage valves is the Starr-Edwards valve. The Bjork-Shiley, St. Jude, and Medtronic valves are examples of the tilting-disk valve. These mechanical valves have the advantage of durability and the disadvantage of being highly thrombogenic and requiring life-long anticoagulation. The tissue valves such as the porcine or the bovine pericardial valve are less thrombogenic but reports of calcification, fibrosis, and leaflet disruption have raised questions about their durability.

## CONGENITAL HEART DISEASE

A wide spectrum of congenital lesions may be seen in adults and the majority can be corrected at low risk(16,17). The long-term morbidity of **large atrial defects** compared with the low operative mortality greatly favors surgical intervention even in mildly symptomatic cases. In individuals with certain forms of cyanotic heart disease, definitive repair can prevent the threat of systemic embolization by closure of right-to-left shunts.

On the other hand, small ventricular septal defects(18) and patent ductus arteriosus(19) are associated with a benign course, and the decision is often made not to operate on these patients despite the low operative morbidity and mortality. The lack of significant surgical improvement in natural history and the relatively high operative morbidity in patients over 35 with **coarctation of the aorta** often leads to the decision to manage these patients with antihypertensive therapy alone(20).

## REFERENCES

1.  McIntosh HD, Garcia JA:  The first decade of aortocoronary bypass grafting, 1967-1977:  A review.  Circulation 57:405, 1978.

2.  Kent KM, Borer JS, Green MV, et al.:  Effects of coronary artery bypass on global and regional left ventricular function during exercise.  N Engl J Med 298:1434, 1978.

3.  European Coronary Surgery Study Group: Long-term results of prospective randomized study of coronary artery bypass surgery in stable angina pectoris.  Lancet 2:1173, 1982.

4.  CASS Principal Investigators and their Associates:  CASS: A randomized trial of coronary artery bypass surgery.  Survival data. Circulation 68:939, 1983.

5.  Takaro T, Hultgren HN, Detre KM, et al.:  The Veterans Administration Cooperative Study of Stable Angina-Current Status. Circulation 65 (suppl II):II-60, 1982.

6.  Hurst JW, King SB, Logue RB:  Value of coronary bypass surgery. Controversies in cardiology:  Part I.  Am J Cardiol 42:308, 1978.

7.  Passamini E, Davis KB, Gillespie MJ, et al.:  A randomized trial of coronary artery bypass surgery.  Survival of patients with a low ejection fraction.  N Engl J Med 312:1665, 1985.

8.  Bonow RO, Kent KM, et al.:  Exercise-induced ischemia in mildly symptomatic patients with coronary artery disease and preserved left ventricular function.  N Engl J Med 311:1339, 1984.

 9.  Kobayashi T, Mendez AM, Zubiate P, et al.:   Repeat aortocoronary bypass grafting.  Early and late results.  Chest 73:445, 1978.

10.  Shark WM, Kass RM:   Repeat myocardial revascularization in coronary disease therapy:   Consideration of primary bypass failures and success of second graft surgery.  Am Heart J 102:303, 1981.

11.  Lytle BW, Loop TD, Cosgrove DM, et al.:   Long term (5 to 12 years) serial studies of internal mammary artery and saphenous vein coronary bypass grafts.  J Thorac Cardiovasc Surg 89:248, 1985.

12.  Rapaport E:  Natural history of aortic and mitral disease.  Am J Cardiol 35:221, 1975.

13.  Rahimtoola SH:  Early valve replacement for preservation of ventricular function.  Am J Cardiol 40:472, 1977.

14.  O'Rourke RA, Crawford MH:  Timing of valve replacement in patients with chronic aortic regurgitation.  Circulation 61:493, 1980 (editorial).

15.  Roberts WC:  Substitute cardiac valves.  Advantages and disadvantages of four commonly used ones.  Adv Cardiol 22:252,1978.

16.  Coles JC, Gargely NF, Buttegliero JB:  Congenital heart disease in the adult.  Arch Surg 89:130, 1964.

17.  Cooley DA, Hallman GL, Hamman AS:  Congenital cardiovascular anomalies in adults.  Result of surgical treatment in 167 patients over 35.  Am J Cardiol 17:303, 1966.

18.  Corone P, Doyon F, Gaudeu S, et al.:  Natural history of ventricular septal defect.  A study involving 790 cases.  Circulation 55:908, 1977.

19.  Campbell M:  Natural history of persistent ductus arteriosus.  Br Heart J 30:4, 1968.

20.  Liberthson RR, Pennington DG, Jacobs ML, et al.:  Coarctation of the aorta:  Review of 234 patients and clarification of management problems.  Am J Cardiol 43:835, 1979.

# Index